Implementing Occupation-centred Practice

This practical text supports occupational therapy students and educators as they navigate the opportunities and challenges of practice learning. Reflecting contemporary and innovative occupation-centred practice, it sets out a step-by-step guide to using this knowledge across a range of settings. The clear structure, templates, examples and strategies it presents demonstrate how contemporary theory can be used to inform and guide practice.

Implementing Occupation-centred Practice is an essential resource for occupational therapy students during their placement preparation and throughout their placement. It also serves as a tool for practice educators who are looking for assistance in structuring learning for their students.

Karina Dancza is Assistant Professor, Health and Social Sciences, at the Singapore Institute of Technology, Singapore.

Sylvia Rodger was Director of Research and Education at the Cooperative Research Centre for Living with Autism, The University of Queensland, Australia.

"Health care is finally focusing on health which creates a major opportunity for occupational therapists who focus on occupational performance (doing), which we know enables participation (engagement), and we know participation contributes to well-being (health and quality of life). Occupational therapists do these things because of their special skill set and occupational lens. This book will support educators and challenge students to understand their unique and powerful role in enabling occupational performance."

Carolyn Baum, Washington University School of Medicine, St. Louis, USA

"For students, this book is a self-guided resource that helps them transfer their knowledge to various practice settings. The guide reminds students that regardless of where they practice, two things constantly influence their interactions with clients: occupation-centred theories and the occupational therapy process. Therefore, the book provides a review of theories centred on occupation and a trove of guided activities for each step of the Occupational Therapy Intervention Process Model (OTIPM). While some students and practice educators may be unfamiliar with the OTIPM specifically, they will be familiar with the process it follows through the stages of occupational therapy assessment, goal setting, intervention and reassessment. The OTIPM lays out the steps of the reasoning and practice process shared by occupational therapists across settings. Therefore, students and educators who may not use the OTIPM per se will still benefit from the book's structure and the self-guided activities that Dr. Dancza has created for each stage of the occupational therapy process."

Barbara Hooper, Colorado State University, USA

Implementing Occupation-centred Practice

A Practical Guide for Occupational Therapy Practice Learning

EDITED BY
KARINA DANCZA AND SYLVIA RODGER

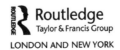

Routledge
Taylor & Francis Group

LONDON AND NEW YORK

First published 2018
by Routledge
2 Park Square, Milton Park, Abingdon, Oxon OX14 4RN

and by Routledge
711 Third Avenue, New York, NY 10017

Routledge is an imprint of the Taylor & Francis Group, an informa business

British Library Cataloguing-in-Publication Data
A catalogue record for this book is available from the British Library

Library of Congress Cataloging-in-Publication Data
Names: Dancza, Karina, editor. | Rodger, Sylvia, editor.
Title: Implementing occupation-centred practice : a practical guide for
   occupational therapy practice learning / edited by Karina Dancza and
   Sylvia Rodger.
Description: Abingdon, Oxon ; New York, NY : Routledge, 2018. | Includes
   bibliographical references and index.
Identifiers: LCCN 2017048528 | ISBN 9781138238466 (hardback) |
   ISBN 9781138238480 (pbk.) | ISBN 9781315297415 (ebook)
Subjects: MESH: Occupational Therapy—methods
Classification: LCC RM735.3 | NLM WB 555 | DDC 615.8/515—dc23
LC record available at https://lccn.loc.gov/2017048528

ISBN: 978-1-138-23846-6 (hbk)
ISBN: 978-1-138-23848-0 (pbk)
ISBN: 978-1-315-29741-5 (ebk)

Typeset in Garamond
by Apex CoVantage, LLC

Visit the eResources: www.routledge.com/9781138238480

For Sylvia
An inspirational thinker, passionate influencer and generous spirit.

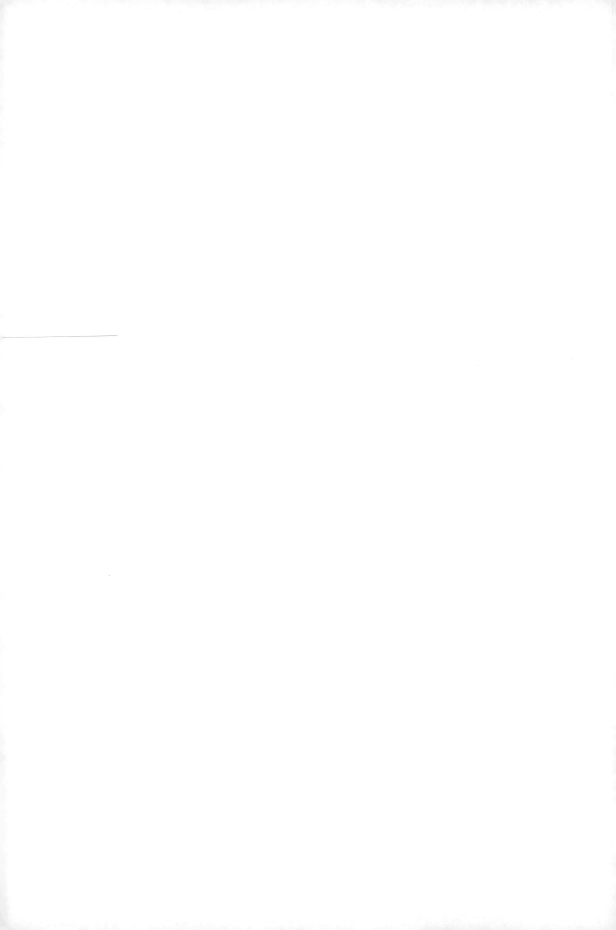

CONTENTS

AUTHOR DETAILS

EDITORS
Editor 1: **Dr. Karina Dancza** PhD, MA(SEN), PGCLT, BAppSc(OT), FHEA
Assistant Professor, Health and Social Sciences
Singapore Institute of Technology
10 Dover Drive, Singapore
kdancza@gmail.com

Editor 2: **Professor Sylvia Rodger** AM., PhD, MEdSt, BOccThy
Emeritus Professor, School of Health and Rehabilitation Sciences
Director Research and Education Cooperative Research Centred for Living with Autism,
The University of Queensland
St Lucia, Brisbane, Queensland, Australia

CHAPTER AUTHORS
Dr. Jodie Copley PhD, BOccThy
Senior Lecturer of Occupational Therapy School of Health and Rehabilitation Sciences
The University of Queensland
St Lucia, Brisbane, Queensland Australia

Sarah E. Cullen MScOT, BA
Case Manager
NeuroHealth Case Management Services
London, United Kingdom

Sarah Harvey MA, PGCAP, BSc(hons)OT, FHEA
Senior Lecturer in Occupational Therapy
School of Allied Health Professions, Faculty of Health and Wellbeing
Canterbury Christ Church University
Canterbury, Kent, United Kingdom

Jeannette Head MSc, PGCLT, DipCOT
Programme Director MSc Health and Wellbeing
Senior Lecturer Centre for Work Based Learning and Continuing Development
Canterbury Christ Church University
Medway, Kent, United Kingdom

Caroline Hui MSc, OT(C), erg.
Pediatric Occupational Therapist
Lecturer and Clinical Supervisor
Université de Sherbrooke
Sherbrooke, Quebec, Canada

Dr. Ann Kennedy-Behr PhD, MOccThy, BAppSc(OT)
Lecturer and Program Coordinator, Bachelor Occupational Therapy (Honours)
School of Health and Sports Sciences, Faculty of Science, Health, Education and
Engineering
University of the Sunshine Coast
Sunshine Coast, Queensland, Australia

Sue Mesa MSc, PGCLT, BSc(hons)OT
Senior Lecturer, School of Health Sciences
York St John University
York, United Kingdom

Dr. Monica Moran DocSocSc, MPhil(OT), PGCert, DipCOT
Associate Professor of Rural Health, WA Centre for Rural Health
University of Western Australia
Western Australia, Australia

Anita Volkert EdD Candidate, PGCLT, BAppSc(OT)
National Manager – Professional Standards and Representation
Occupational Therapy Australia
Melbourne, Victoria, Australia

FOREWORDS

I write this foreword at the request of Dr. Karina Dancza shortly after the death of my dear, dear friend Sylvia Rodger. I am honoured to do so because I know and have been a beneficiary of the passion which Sylvia had for occupational therapists to gain the understanding that they have a unique and special skill to go beyond the medical issues managed by physicians and the movement issues managed by physical therapists. She always challenged occupational therapists to use their knowledge of the factors that support and influence people's capacity to do and modelled that the occupational therapist must have the skills and knowledge, and use a professional process, to enable people to do what they want and need to do to live their lives. This book is designed to help students bring their practice into focus; the content is presented as stages of their practice learning.

Occupational therapists are leading the changes in health care (as example, the work of Dr. Rodger in leading and addressing the clinical and research issues of children with autism across the biomedical and sociocultural levels of care) and have the opportunity to take major roles in helping people achieve health and well-being. Occupational therapists are ideally situated to respond to the changing delivery of healthcare, where we are experiencing shifts from a treatment-only approach to one where the value of primary and secondary prevention is recognised. Occupational therapists are critical in supporting people as they age or transition from one developmental stage to another or face the consequences of managing chronic disease and disability. Every occupational therapist has the opportunity to use his/her knowledge to improve occupational lives.

Being an agent of change requires clinicians to have a well-developed approach to use their unique capabilities as clinicians addressing the emerging opportunities for the changing health care system. Health care is finally focusing on health, which creates a major opportunity for occupational therapists who focus on occupational performance (doing), which we know enables participation (engagement) and we know participation contributes to well-being (health and quality of life). We see these changes when effort is placed on building safe communities, helping people age in place and prevent falls, transition programs to engage teenagers with disabilities in pre-work and eventually worker roles, addressing the issues that help people avoid re-hospitalization. Occupational therapists do these things because of their special skill set and occupational lens. This book will support educators and challenge students to understand their unique and powerful role in enabling occupational performance.

Carolyn Baum, PhD, OTR/L, FAOTA
Elias Michael Director and Professor of Occupational
Therapy, Neurology and Social Work
Washington University School of Medicine, St. Louis MO

****

Research and resources that benefit students and educators often arise from struggles encountered in practice. I learned that this dynamic was the back story of Dr. Karina Dancza's *Implementing occupation-centred practice: a practical guide for occupational therapy practice learning*. Dr. Dancza was a practice educator in a role-emerging setting, a setting without clear roles for occupational therapy and no occupational therapist. She found few resources to guide her work with students, to help them chart a path that reflected the distinct value of occupational therapy. "I wasn't sure where to start," Dr. Dancza shared. On-site personnel helped students with logistics but no one was there on a daily basis to guide their identity formation and competence as *occupational* therapists. In spite of limited resources, Dr. Dancza met weekly with students and listened to their practice stories and dilemmas. She innovated solutions, ways to address dilemmas, and how to connect students' coursework to their experiences.

But something was missing. Without being on site with students when situations happened, Dr. Dancza puzzled over how to help them reason, make connections to coursework and support their development as occupation-based practitioners. As Dancza explained, "I couldn't find a book, any resource, that could reinforce what I was telling students – a resource they could use when I was not around." She rolled up her sleeves and got to work collaborating with students and other practitioners to create the educational intervention she was looking for, which ultimately culminated in this book. She and the students wrote down what worked to support them as novice occupation-based practitioners. Dr. Dancza sent what they wrote to other practice educators and students in role-emerging and in role-established practice sites such as acute care and rehabilitation. She collected data from all those students and therapists who used the book. Through many rounds of testing and revision, Dr. Dancza created *Implementing occupation-centred practice: a practical guide for occupational therapy practice learning* for students muddling through sites where they are largely self-directed. However, in creating this book for students and educators in one setting, she provided a resource for all students on practice education and their educators. Her hope was to provide a resource so that "practice educators do not have to start from scratch." Perhaps if more practice educators have resources like this book they will feel less alone and better equipped to guide students through the elements of occupation-based practice in both role-emerging and role-established practice sites, ultimately serving broader populations of people with occupational challenges.

For students, this book is a self-guided resource that helps them transfer their knowledge to various practice settings. The guide reminds students that regardless of where they practice, two things constantly influence their interactions with clients: occupation-centred theories and the occupational therapy process. Therefore, the book provides a review of theories centred on occupation and a trove of guided activities for each step of the Occupational Therapy Intervention Process Model (OTIPM) (Fisher, 2009). While some students and practice educators may be unfamiliar with the OTIPM specifically, they will be familiar with the process it follows through the stages of occupational therapy assessment, goal setting, intervention and reassessment. The OTIPM lays out the steps of the reasoning and practice process shared by occupational therapists across settings. Therefore, students and educators who may not use the OTIPM per se will still benefit from the book's structure based on the OTIPM and the self-guided activities that Dr. Dancza has created for each stage of the occupational therapy process.

As a self-guided resource, the book conveys to students that they are in charge of their learning; therefore, they must be intentional about bridging coursework to the practice environment and must centre learning and practice on occupation. Further, since the book sets up the student as a self-directed learner, students will benefit from the review of learning theories in Chapter 14. That is, if students are in charge of their learning, then they need to understand how learning works and intentionally apply learning theory to their own self-directed learning tasks.

For practice educators, this book assists in setting up practice education experiences, including a helpful overview of learning theories that undergird such experiences. But the book also addresses two common, yet seldom discussed, challenges for practice educators: the challenge of remembering the state of their knowledge when they, too, were an almost-but-not-yet therapist; and the challenge of realizing how the knowledge from those novice years still informs practice even if that knowledge is no longer explicitly available because it has become so ingrained in what they do each day. This book helps experts remember that novices need repeatedly to apply theory to practice, walk through the steps of the occupational therapy process, talk with clients about occupation, watch clients engage in occupation, discern the causes of clients' difficulties, break down tasks to support client engagement, teach clients how to perform tasks and perform many other novice skills. Each activity students complete in this book simultaneously reminds educators what students at this level need to learn and the kinds of learning activities educators may create for students in the contexts of their own settings.

As an educator and education researcher, I am also interested in creating profession-specific education resources. Like Dr. Dancza, my research arose from struggles encountered in practice and finding limited resources to address those struggles. Specifically, I found few resources to help me implement occupation-centred education; that is, education that links all topics and practice skills to the field's central focus on helping people become and remain meaningfully occupied. Like Dr. Dancza, I rolled up my sleeves and went to work creating the resources I was lacking. In studying occupational therapy education, I have seen that academic educators can teach topics and skills disconnected from the profession's central focus on occupation. When this happens, it is believed that students consequently struggle to grasp their distinctive contributions to health and social care. Similarly, practice educators and their students can get overly focused on the skills that are prominent in their specific practice setting, forgetting to circle back and explicitly link those skills to occupation which is at the heart of the occupational therapy reasoning process. Dr. Dancza's book seeks to remind educators and students alike to make those links explicit – because ultimately, occupational therapy's distinct contributions lie in how setting-specific skills and processes are actively linked back to the profession's aim of enabling occupation.

Barbara Hooper, Ph.D., OTR, FAOTA
Associate Professor
Academic Program Director
Colorado State University, USA

REFERENCE

Fisher AG (2009) *Occupational therapy intervention process model: A model for planning and implementing top-down, client centred, and occupation-based interventions.* Fort Collins, CO: Three Star Press.

ACKNOWLEDGEMENTS

I am grateful to all of those with whom I have had the pleasure to work during my doctoral research and writing this book. The contributions, guidance and enthusiasm of the students, academics, practice learning staff members and clients have made this project possible.

I would like to express my gratitude to my colleagues from Canterbury Christ Church University and The University of Queensland, who gave me the opportunity to pursue my passion. Also to the staff members at Routledge for their assistance and responsiveness to the many questions that were put to them.

I acknowledge the work of Professor Anne G. Fisher, whose occupation-centred vision has inspired my own occupational therapy practice.

I would like to thank the team of expert writers and reviewers, who have selflessly contributed their time and energy to the development of this book.

Thanks are also due to Associate Professor Monica Moran and Associate Professor Louise Farnworth, both of whom stepped in and supported me over the final hurdles.

I would like to thank my family, friends and especially my husband Viktor and my father John Temme, for their love and belief in me.

Finally, I am indebted to my co-editor, mentor and friend Professor Sylvia Rodger. You will be forever remembered.

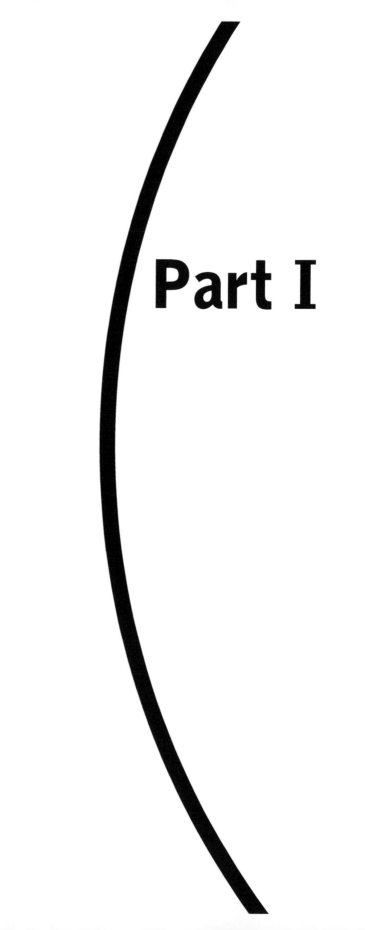

Part I

FOUNDATIONS OF OCCUPATION-CENTRED PRACTICE

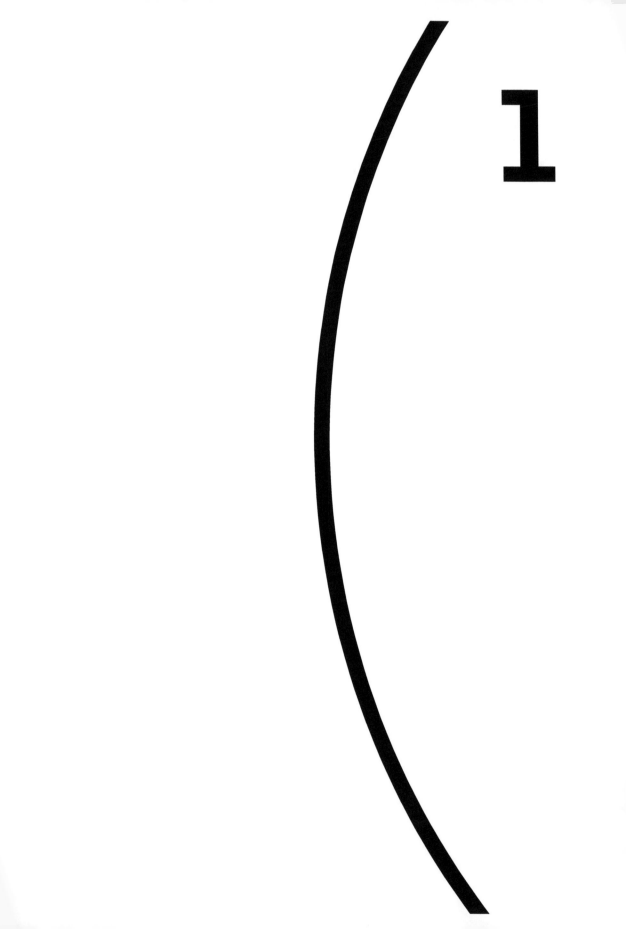

1

CHAPTER 1
GUIDE TO THE BOOK
Karina Dancza

Occupational therapy is about the creation of health through the vital human need to be occupied (Hooper, 2006). Within occupational therapy education, students and educators explore the relationship between occupation, health and well-being. On the surface this relationship may seem to be straightforward, but when we apply these concepts in real-life situations we discover them as troublesome, changeable and filled with contradictions and tensions.

Implementing occupation-centred practice: a practical guide for occupational therapy practice learning supports the application of contemporary theory about the relationship between health and well-being to the practice of occupational therapy. Learning through doing is promoted in this step-by-step guidance for today's occupational therapy students and educators (supervisors).

The idea for this book developed within my own practice as an occupational therapy educator. I was conscious of wanting to support occupational therapy students consolidate their understanding of occupation and its value for health and well-being during their practice learning experiences (placements). In doing this, however, I found that applying an 'occupation-centred' perspective was indeed troublesome, changeable and filled with contradictions and tensions.

From this place of discomfort I embarked on my doctoral research investigating student learning of occupation-centred practice (Dancza, 2015). Five years and four action research cycles later, I was much better informed about how students learn in practice and what supports and challenges this learning. This book was born out of these experiences and the collaborations with students and educators, both within my own university in the United Kingdom and my colleagues internationally. I am particularly grateful to my co-editor, supervisor, mentor and friend Professor Sylvia Rodger, without whom I would never have started or persisted on this journey.

Practice learning takes many forms. In this book we have illustrated how concepts and strategies about occupation-centred practice can be applied within established occupational therapy services and occupational therapy roles which are in new areas of practice (role-emerging or project areas). While many aspects apply in all placement structures, at times there are differences which we will consider separately.

To present a little certainly within the troublesome and changeable context of practice learning, this book offers students and educators a coherent occupational therapy process from beginning to end. At times this might seem prescriptive, particularly when we explore the use of occupational performance analysis as a key assessment tool and a way to structure our professional reasoning and reporting. Our experience has shown that when students are learning about these important concepts they need a firm foundation which they can logically follow. Without a firm foundation, it is more difficult for students to appropriately select which theories and tools to use. However, once they feel confident in an occupational therapy process they can adapt, change and deviate from this foundation as their understanding develops.

The book is presented in three parts, each with a different focus:

- Part I outlines our contemporary understanding of occupation-centred practice and presents reminders of some of our occupational therapy models. We then present the 'engine house' of occupational therapy with the key tools of occupational profiling, activity and occupational performance analysis, including practical templates and examples. This section is designed to help students and educators develop a collective understanding of what it means to practice in an occupation-centred way.
- Part II uses the Occupational Therapy Intervention Process Model (OTIPM: Fisher, 2009) and practical examples to guide students and educators through each stage of the occupational therapy process. The OTIPM (Fisher, 2009) was selected as it has a clear and consistent focus on occupation in each step of the process. This model can be used with other occupational therapy models, which is important as students and practice areas often use a range of resources. Educators are encouraged to support students contextualise the information to their own practice learning contexts as this is critical in supporting students' learning. Key areas which benefit from contextualisation are summarised in Appendix 1.1 and referenced as 'educator examples here' and indicated by this image throughout Part II.
- Part III is focused on supporting educators in their role as supervisors. We commence this section with a demonstration of how educational theory can help us understand practice learning and develop enriched learning opportunities. We then use six case study examples of the implementation of this book from across established and non-established occupational therapy practice learning settings. It is based on examples shared by educators who have used a draft of this book in their own supervision with occupational therapy students. These case studies offer fascinating insights into the successes and challenges of practice learning, with practical tips for making the most of these experiences. Moreover, illustrated in Part III is how the OTIPM (Fisher, 2009) can be used successfully even if it is less well known to students or educators.

As you may see from the overview, this book is intended to support both students and educators. The Part I chapters are relevant for both students and educators as they offer foundation knowledge to create a shared understanding of occupation-centred occupational therapy. Part II focuses mainly on students with the step-by-step guide to practice learning. However, suggestions are also presented for educators to support their guidance of students throughout the occupational therapy process. Part III is written with the educator in mind. It offers an introduction to educational theories applied in occupational therapy practice learning and provides examples through case study illustrations. All chapters are, however, not exclusive to students or educators. Having both educator and student 'on the same page' can support understanding of each other's perspectives. Using the book in supervision discussions can help maintain a clear focus for all involved.

To support occupational therapy students and educators navigate practice learning opportunities, this book is enhanced with learning features to reinforce understanding of key topics. There is a Glossary (beginning on p. 293) which outlines how we will use terms throughout this book. We have attempted to include synonyms as we are aware of the array of terms used internationally to describe practice learning. Additional features of this book to look out for include:

Intended chapter outcomes		These intended chapter outcomes offer a summary of what you will learn within the chapter.
	Stage in the OTIPM	In Part II, each chapter begins with a highlighted diagram of the OTIPM which indicates where we are in the occupational therapy process.
	Activity	Throughout the book there are suggested activities (indicated by images such as those shown here) which are designed to support students consolidate their learning of the topics covered in the section.

|  | Educator examples here | We have also pointed out throughout the book where we think it is helpful for educators to offer specific suggestions or examples to students about their own practice context. These are indicated by the 'educator examples here' and image and are summarised in Appendix 1.1. |
| Chapter summary | | Each chapter concludes with a summary of the main points discussed to help reinforce learning. |

We hope that you will find this book useful, interesting and challenging as you navigate practice learning opportunities as a student, educator or practitioner. Occupational therapy has much to offer society. Through making the most of our understanding of occupation and its relationship to health and well-being, we can as a profession continue to be a positive influence and agents of change in our communities.

APPENDIX 1.1

'EDUCATOR EXAMPLES HERE' SUMMARY

Place in this book	Topic	Suggested information
Chapter 5 (p. 85)	Recommended preliminary reading	Books, articles, websites etc. which illustrate the role of occupational therapy within a similar workplace context
Chapter 5 (p. 87)	Introducing yourself	Examples or key points that student(s) need to be aware of in explaining their role in this context

Place in this book	Topic	Suggested information
Chapter 5 (p. 93)	Placement timeline	An outline of the number of days / weeks of placement and how the student(s) are expected to progress during this time
Chapter 7 (p. 118)	Questions for establishing priorities	Questions to help students establish priority areas with the people they are working with
Chapter 8 (p. 131)	Risk assessment	Risk assessment templates or tools which are relevant for this context
Chapter 8 (p. 138)	Assessment tools	Assessment tools or materials which the student(s) may come across during the placement
Chapter 9 (p. 148)	Progress notes	Progress notes format and/ or examples
Chapter 9 (p. 150)	Reports	Report format and/or examples
Chapter 10 (p. 174)	Goal setting tools	Tools or materials used in the setting to help determine client goals
Chapter 10 (p. 178)	Goals	Goal setting structure and/or examples
Chapter 12 (p. 204)	Compensatory intervention approaches	Resources or ideas for compensatory interventions relevant for the setting
Chapter 12 (p. 205)	Education-based intervention approaches	Resources or ideas for education-based interventions relevant for the setting
Chapter 12 (p. 207)	Skills-based intervention approaches	Resources or ideas for skills-based interventions relevant for the setting
Chapter 12 (p. 208)	Restorative intervention approaches	Resources or ideas for restorative interventions relevant for the setting
Chapter 13 (p. 223)	Evaluation tools	Evaluation tools or materials which the student(s) may come across during placement

REFERENCES

Dancza KM (2015) *Structure and uncertainty: The 'just right' balance for occupational therapy student learning on role-emerging placements in schools.* Doctor of Philosophy, The University of Queensland, Queensland, Australia.

Fisher AG (2009) *Occupational therapy intervention process model: A model for planning and implementing top-down, client centred, and occupation-based interventions.* Fort Collins, CO: Three Star Press.

Hooper B (2006) 'Epistemological transformation in occupational therapy: Educational implications and challenges'. *OTJR: Occupation, Participation and Health, 26*(1), 15–24.

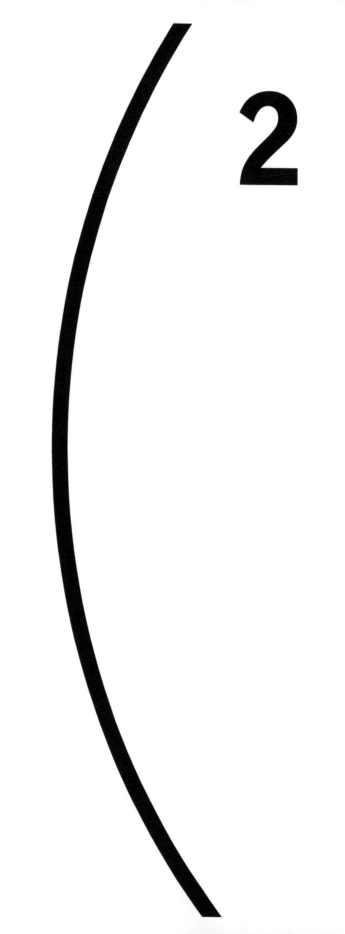

2

CHAPTER 2
OCCUPATION-CENTRED PRACTICE AND REASONING
Karina Dancza and Sylvia Rodger

INTENDED CHAPTER OUTCOMES

By the end of this chapter, readers will have an overview of:

– The unique occupation-centred perspective of occupational therapy
– The difference between occupation-focused and occupation-based practice as a way of reflecting on occupational therapy services
– How close or far away is occupation to practice and the implications of this for professional identity
– Reasoning including top-down, bottom-up and top-to-bottom-up

INTRODUCTION

In this chapter, we provide an overview of what it is to be an occupational therapist. We begin by offering some ideas about how to reinforce our professional identity (how *occupation* impacts health and well-being) and how to market the value of occupational therapy to the public as well as those who fund our services.

We consider types of reasoning that occupational therapists use such as top-down and bottom-up reasoning, the former being more occupation-centred (Fisher, 2009). We then explore occupation-centred practice as an overarching term, and how occupation-focused and occupation-based practice fits within this (Fisher, 2013). Next, we address practice from the perspective of how close or distant occupation is to the therapist's thinking. Finally, we discuss how occupation-centred practice relates to participation.

DEFINING OCCUPATIONAL THERAPY

It is not uncommon when meeting a new person that they ask you what it is that you do. As occupational therapists, we understand how influential a work role is to our own identity. Why is it then, that when asked to explain what it is that an occupational therapist does, many of us are filled with dread?

We may stumble about an explanation which can turn into a lengthy monologue describing many of the tasks that we carry out within our work (such as helping an elderly person to get home from hospital following a fall, working with a child to ride his/her bike or adjusting the environment so that a person can return to work following a brain injury). We may state or imply that occupational therapy is different in different settings, as it is such a diverse profession. We may also avoid the use of the word *occupation* as it can cause confusion with people thinking our work has something to do with either employment services or occupational health and safety. Issues may be magnified when we abbreviate our name to 'OT': *at best, we distance ourselves from occupation;* at worst, we are confused with other acronyms like *over-time, operating theatre* or even *information technology* (as OT can be misheard as IT!).

Having an ambiguous explanation of our role creates significant challenges for us as a profession. An overly long and complicated explanation encourages our audience to tune-out to the principal elements of our role. Suggesting we are different in different settings emphasises a lack of cohesion and common thread between us, adding to role blurring and a devaluing of our core philosophy. By not using the word 'occupation,' we are also missing an important opportunity to market ourselves and link what we do with our professional title.

Coming up with a short, simple, yet comprehensive definition of occupational therapy is challenging, yet essential for the continuing prosperity of the profession. Our offer has been adapted from World Federation of Occupational Therapists (2012) and the Royal College of Occupational Therapists (2015a): "Occupational therapists are concerned with how people 'occupy' their time."

Figure 2.1 illustrates this explanation. We might expand by saying:

> "What people do to *occupy* their time (their occupations) is fundamental to their health and well-being. Daily life is made up of many *occupations*, such as getting ready to go out, cooking a meal or working. An occupational therapist will help people who may need support or advice if they are not able to do their occupations due to illness, disability, circumstances or because of changes in their lives as they get older."

Finding an explanation of occupational therapy that works for you is important. It is critical, however, that we as a profession agree on common elements to our explanations. If all occupational therapists *link the importance of occupation with health and well-being* as the primary focus of the profession, it will provide a common identity for us, regardless of where and with whom we work.

Using the word 'occupation' with a simple explanation of what we mean, can also promote the link between our name and what we do. Our language is constantly evolving which is evidenced by the everyday use and understanding of several 'made up' words (e.g. Google – meaning an internet search engine; Twitter – a social media site). Branding ourselves clearly using *occupation* is more likely to support the community's understanding

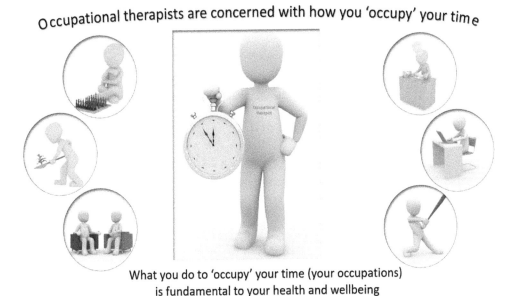

Occupational therapists are concerned with how you 'occupy' your time

What you do to 'occupy' your time (your occupations)
is fundamental to your health and wellbeing

Figure 2.1 Explaining occupational therapy

of our profession. Similarly, using the full title of occupational therapist rather than shortening it to 'OT' may further support the promotion of our profession.

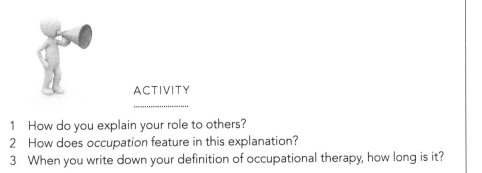

ACTIVITY
....

1   How do you explain your role to others?
2   How does *occupation* feature in this explanation?
3   When you write down your definition of occupational therapy, how long is it?

THE IMPORTANCE OF OCCUPATION

The Royal College of Occupational Therapists (the professional body in the United Kingdom) released a position statement (2015a) which emphasised the importance of occupation to health and well-being and the role of the occupational therapist in promoting occupation. In this document, it was stated that:

Occupation should be considered a basic need and human right, like eating, drinking and breathing (Dunton, 1919). There is a renewed understanding of how engagement in occupation is therapy and fundamental to health and wellbeing (Wilcock, 2006). . . . The focus of the practitioner in any setting, with any service user group is to maximise occupational performance and participation.

Importantly, humans are occupational beings and are experts on their own occupations. Additionally, Townsend and Polatajko (2007) outlined several other core beliefs about occupation:

- It organises human behaviour.
- It develops and changes over a lifetime.
- It shapes and is shaped by the environment.
- It has therapeutic potential.

Occupations give meaning to life (Townsend and Polatajko, 2007). Occupation should not be considered part of a person's life only if it is easy to do, or if services have time to focus on it. The Royal College of Occupational Therapists' position statement reinforces that occupational therapists' primary focus is occupation. If the duties of an occupational therapist also include generic health and human care tasks, then they should not be undertaken at the expense of assisting clients to engage in occupations. Occupational therapists are educated in the fundamentals of occupation, drawing from occupational science, and these skills and expertise should be front and centre of our practice and must not be side-lined when resources are stretched.

Occupation-centred practice means that occupation is at the core of everything that we do. We believe that it is through occupation that health and well-being (Wilcock, 2006) and justice (Townsend and Polatajko, 2007) are influenced.

This is a unique perspective from that of many other professionals, as it is often the body functions and structures (e.g. memory, cognition, motor, perceptual or sensory abilities and skills – see the International Classification of Functioning, Disability and Health in Chapter 3, Figure 3.1) which are the close focus of their interventions. It is anticipated that improvements in body functions and structures will lead to improvements in occupation and participation. However, evidence is limited which suggests that interventions focused at one level (e.g. body functions and structures) translate to improvements at another level (e.g. occupation and participation) (Novak et al., 2013). Therefore, if you want to see improvements, your interventions need to focus on occupation and participation. It may also be that through engaging in one's occupations, body functions and structures change. However, these changes are a bonus rather than our primary focus.

There is growing evidence regarding the benefits of using an occupation-centred approach with children and adults who experience a range of occupational performance challenges. Practicing from an occupation-centred perspective has also shown improvements in job satisfaction for occupational therapists as it aligns with our profession's unique perspective (Estes and Pierce, 2012).

UNPACKING REASONING: TOP-DOWN, BOTTOM-UP, TOP-TO-BOTTOM-UP

Reasoning is a "context dependent way of thinking and decision making in professional practice to guide practice actions" (Higgs and Jones, 2008, p. 4). Reasoning is used throughout the occupational therapy process from the preliminary stages of information gathering (what information should be sought and from whom?), goal setting and prioritising, making decisions about assessment, intervention and what and how to re-evaluate a client's performance. There are many classifications of reasoning that have been proposed by various authors (e.g., Mattingly and Fleming, 1994; Schell and Cervero, 1993; Taylor, 2008) at various times (see Chapter 11).

The more experienced the occupational therapist is in an area of practice, the more automatic or subconscious his/her reasoning becomes. Being occupation-centred means that occupation remains core at all stages of the occupational therapy process. This can sound obvious, but there are common patterns of reasoning which can be thought of as occupation-centred, but in reality, their focus is elsewhere. Fisher (2009) described three categories of reasoning within practice – namely top-down, bottom-up and top-to-bottom-up reasoning – that will be expanded upon here.

TOP-DOWN REASONING

Top-down reasoning (Fisher, 2009) can be considered as the reasoning used when engaged in occupation-centred practice. Within the occupational therapy process, it has key stages that are identified in Figure 2.2.

These stages involve an identification of the client's occupational needs, assessment of these needs (i.e., occupation-focused and occupation-based analysis), intervention which is designed to enable performance of that occupation and evaluation of success through improvement in performance of this occupation. A more detailed explanation of top-down reasoning is given in the Occupational Therapy Intervention Process Model (Fisher, 2009) in Chapter 3, which is the basis for the process described in Part II of this book.

BOTTOM-UP REASONING

Bottom-up reasoning (Fisher, 2009) is commonly associated with a medical perspective of the person. Bottom-up reasoning begins with an assessment of the underlying body functions and structures (e.g., gross and fine motor skills, strength, sensory, posture, joint range of motion, visual perception, memory, anxiety, depression, cognition etc.). When strengths and impairments are identified, assumptions are made about how this might impact on various occupations (e.g., cooking, shopping, going to work etc.). Intervention often involves a focus on restoring, repairing or developing the body functions and structures which are felt to be impeding occupational performance (e.g. strengthening

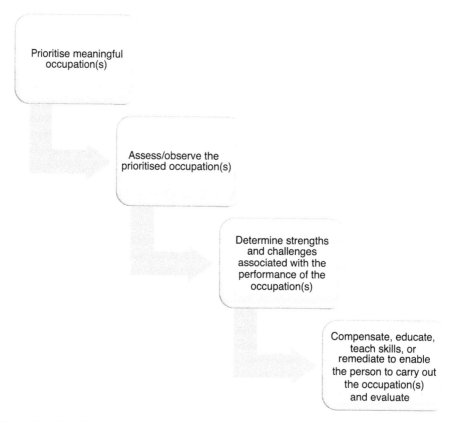

Figure 2.2 Top-down reasoning
Adapted from Fisher (2009).

exercises, memory games, self-esteem groups, relaxation techniques). Evaluation focuses on any improvement in the underlying body functions and structures using specific assessments of these functions, rather than the impact on occupations. This is illustrated in Figure 2.3.

TOP-TO-BOTTOM-UP REASONING

Top-to-bottom-up reasoning (Fisher, 2009) is a variation on bottom-up reasoning, but can be quite confusing as it attempts to also focus on occupation. As with bottom-up reasoning, this cannot be considered a form of occupation-centred reasoning. The occupational therapist is still placing body functions and structures as central.

Top-to-bottom-up reasoning begins with a focus on the occupations which are important or needed for the person (e.g. an occupation-focused interview). This then jumps to an investigation of the underlying body functions and structures which make up these valued occupations (like motor skills, perception, cognition etc.). Assumptions are made as to how the client's strengths and impairments relate to his/her important occupations, and interventions are chosen that focus on remediating these impairments. Evaluation may

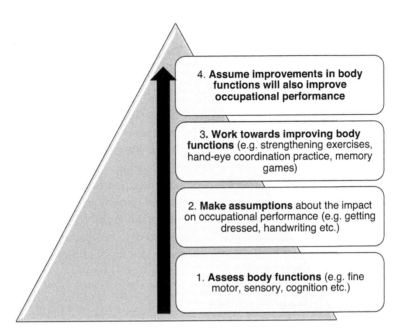

Figure 2.3 Bottom-up reasoning
Adapted from Fisher (2009).

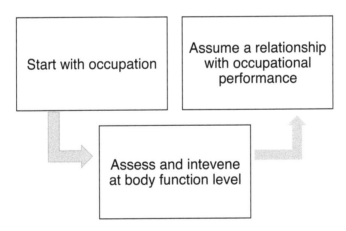

Figure 2.4 Top-to-bottom-up reasoning
Adapted from Fisher (2009).

consider changes in the underlying impairment and/or occupational performance. This is represented in Figure 2.4.

In this book we focus on top-down or occupation-centred reasoning. It is useful, however, to identify when other forms of reasoning are guiding practice areas. Labelling our reasoning correctly will support us to understand the effective elements of our practice and use research evidence appropriately.

REFLECTING ON PRACTICE: OCCUPATION-CENTRED, OCCUPATION-FOCUSED, OCCUPATION-BASED

Top-down reasoning in this book is considered occupation-centred. The Royal College of Occupational Therapists produced further explanation of occupation-centred practice in their briefing of the same name (2015b). In this document, they emphasised the need for occupational therapists to have a common language of what is meant by the terms occupation-centred, occupation-focused and occupation-based (based on the work of Fisher, 2013). Reflecting on practice with these terms in mind, can offer us as occupational therapists a way of critiquing what we are doing and offer some clarity to our professional reasoning processes. Fisher (2013) explains that 'occupation-centred practice' is the overarching term which incorporates occupation-focused and occupation-based elements. This is illustrated in Figure 2.5.

OCCUPATION-FOCUSED PRACTICE

In the occupational therapy process, when you talk about occupations with your client/family/community, this is considered *occupation-focused* (Fisher, 2013). For example, an interview is occupation-focused when you ask about the occupations which are important and make up a person's daily routine. Questions you might ask include "tell me about your typical day/week?", "what can you manage and what are you finding challenging to do?" These discussions enable us to understand the occupational profile (American Occupational Therapy Association, 2014;

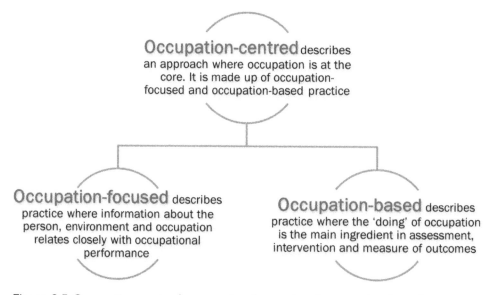

Figure 2.5 Occupation-centred, occupation-focused and occupation-based
Adapted from Fisher (2013).

see Chapter 4) of the person/family/community and helps frame the remainder of occupational therapy involvement.

For discussions to be called 'occupation-focused,' *occupation remains close to the discussion* – that is, how illness, life events and the environment impact on occupation. For example, how a mother's depression might be impacting on her ability to get her children ready for school in the morning. In contrast, if you ask about the person's condition (e.g., depression) or body functions (e.g. mood/anxiety/memory), your conversation has become condition- or body-function focused. Likewise, asking solely about the environment (e.g., does the person have stairs in the home, or a bath or shower) becomes environment-focused. While these different foci may be important at various times, do not confuse them with an occupation focus.

ACTIVITY
....

Think about a person (client) you (or a supervisor) have worked with. Consider the conversations you have had (or witnessed). What elements and percentage of this conversation were:

- Occupation-focused?
- Body function/condition focused?
- Environment-focused?
- Another focus?

It is important for occupational therapists to gather information about a range of areas (such as the person, occupations and environment). Considering the amount of time spent talking about occupation or other areas could offer a point of reflection. Similarly, considering when we introduce the term 'occupation' to our clients may help us to frame our interactions with them and help to explain our role to them. For example, is occupation the first thing you discuss with a client? Or do you talk about occupation during or towards the end of your conversation? Introducing occupation first may help those we work with better understand our focus and role, as well as what to expect from their engagement with occupational therapists.

It is not only our conversations which need to be occupation-focused; our documentation such as reports, progress notes and marketing materials (e.g. website, leaflet or handouts) also promote what it is that we do. Using the language of occupation and relevant examples to provide explanations can influence what others learn about our unique role.

ACTIVITY
....

Have a browse of your service's website or a local occupational therapy service's website. Consider:

– Is there a clear message that occupational therapists are concerned with occupation?
– Does it use the language of occupation (e.g. getting dressed, returning to work, engaging in school etc.)?
– Are there any areas which might be considered confusing for the public about the core focus of occupational therapy?

OCCUPATION-BASED PRACTICE

Occupation-based practice refers to where the *doing* of occupation is at the core of practice (Fisher, 2013). For example, an occupation-based assessment consists of the person doing an occupation (such as a person making a cup of tea in his/her home). Similarly, an occupation-based intervention may adapt/change the way the person is doing specific tasks to improve performance or independence (such as providing a piece of equipment or memory prompts as part of the task sequence). Finally, evaluation measures how the person is now doing his/her occupation (for example, can they make a cup of tea independently when they want to?) (Royal College of Occupational Therapists, 2015b).

Occupational therapists have many strategies to enable a person to do his/her occupations. For example, we can break down the activity through activity analysis (see Chapter 4) and grade and/or adapt elements of the activity to support the person to improve his/ her performance. Techniques such as the Cognitive Orientation to daily Occupational Performance (CO-OP; Rodger and Polatajko, 2017) and Occupational Performance Coaching (Graham, Rodger and Kennedy-Behr, 2017) are examples of occupation-based intervention approaches. These consider the person doing an occupation and uses enabling strategies to enhance that performance.

Occupation-based practice should not be confused with the use of assessment techniques where the purpose is to evaluate body functions. For example, a person may be cooking a meal (an occupation). If the occupational therapist is concerned with how a client is cooking a meal so that he/she can enhance the way the client is cooking safely and independently, then this could be considered occupation-based. If, however, the purpose of the cooking observation is for the occupational therapist to assess the person's memory, balance, sequencing, muscle strength etc., then the assessment activity is less occupation-based and more body-function focussed.

While it may be that the person's body functions are impacting on what they are doing (such as a person may forget where the cups are kept when making tea), you cannot 'see' these body functions. You are making assumptions that it is the poor memory, but what you *see* is the person looking in different places for the cups and a slowness to complete the task.

Making assumptions whilst observing can mean that other reasons for the challenges are missed (such as the cups may have been moved recently or the person is unfamiliar with the hospital kitchen). You may also make assumptions that the person's memory might be poor during other activities (such as getting dressed or going shopping), but this does not take into consideration that the activity and environment have changed, so the person's performance is also going to change (thinking about the Person-Environment-Occupation Model, Law et al., 1996, see Chapter 3).

Being occupation-based means that you analyse the person's performance during an observation of him/her doing an occupation, such as cooking a meal. This may reveal a range of points of performance break down, such as a slowness to complete the activity, disorganisation of the kitchen, increased effort when lifting pans or carrying items or an inefficient sequencing of the activity steps. These points of performance breakdown alert the occupational therapist to strategies that might assist the person to carry out the task more efficiently and safely. The intervention occurs while the person conducts the activity and strategies are developed to support them to cook their meal. This may involve grading the activity to make it simpler, changing something in the environment, introducing equipment or teaching skills associated with cooking the meal. This contrasts with attempting to improve the body functions first, such as engaging them in a range of memory games or sequencing activities that have nothing to do with cooking.

ACTIVITY
....

Think again about a person you (or a supervisor) have worked with. Consider what took place in your interaction with that person. What elements of intervention were:

- Occupation-based?
- Environment-based?
- Body-function/structure based?
- Had a different basis?

THE CLOSENESS OF OCCUPATION TO PRACTICE

If you practice in a way which is occupation-centred (capturing elements of occupation-focused and occupation-based practice), then you inevitably remain very close to the person's occupations. If, however, your focus shifts from occupation (handwriting for homework) to preparatory activities (squeezing therapy putty, rubber band finger games) before doing an occupation, then your practice becomes more distant from occupation (and uses top-to-bottom-up reasoning). Figure 2.6 illustrates this continuum.

It could be argued that all health care professionals are focused on enabling people to do their occupations so that they can participate fully in their lives. For example, a doctor may be focused on symptom reduction (e.g. pain) or cure related to a body function or structure (e.g. shoulder surgery), so that the person is well enough to participate in his/her life roles such as golfer or home handyperson (bottom-up reasoning). A physiotherapist may wish to improve walking and works on lower-limb muscle strength training, so that the person can use stairs at home to undertake his/her daily life tasks (top-to-bottom-up reasoning). Therefore, the *ultimate aim* for all health care professionals is to enable people to live their lives.

What makes occupational therapists different is that their *primary and close focus* is occupation (i.e. doing occupations is seen within their practice). We understand that it is important for a person to develop or maintain his/her occupations for health and well-being.

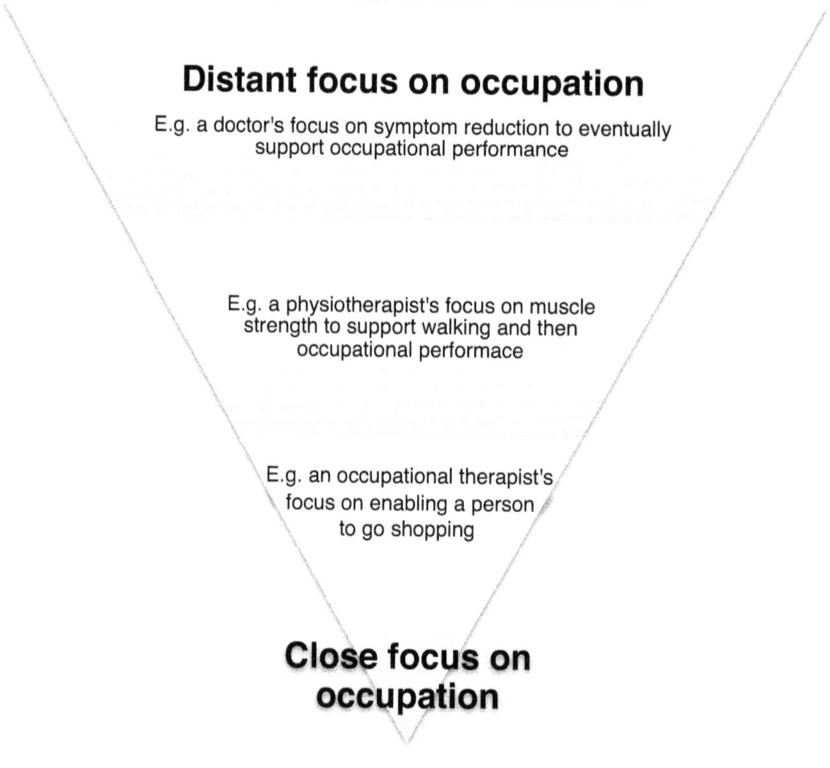

Distant focus on occupation

E.g. a doctor's focus on symptom reduction to eventually
support occupational performance

E.g. a physiotherapist's focus on muscle
strength to support walking and then
occupational performace

E.g. an occupational therapist's
focus on enabling a person
to go shopping

**Close focus on
occupation**

Figure 2.6 Distant and close focus on occupation by various professions

When occupational therapists move away from occupation to focus on developing or maintaining a body function (e.g. squeezing therapy putty, playing rubber band finger games), then their role may overlap and be indistinguishable from that of other professionals.

For example, after Colin had a stroke that left him with right-side weakness and sensory loss, he became increasingly anxious about not being able to keep his financial affairs up-to-date because he needed to be able to sign cheques to pay his bills. His previous therapist had him use an exercise book and practice lines of meaningless loops and circles such as ⌀⌀⌀⌀⌀⌀⌀⌀⌀⌀, ℯℯℯℯℯℯℯℯℯℯ, ∽∽∽∽∽∽, ⦀⦀⦀⦀⦀⦀, ℓℓℓℓℓℓℓ etc. He felt frustrated by this repetition and the childish nature of this preparatory handwriting activity.

There are many ways of paying bills. However, Colin's usual method was writing cheques and he was anxious about using electronic banking. As a first step, the new occupational therapist and Colin decided to work on his cheque writing, but also begin to investigate electronic banking options. The occupational therapist helped him to learn to sign his name by practicing his signature with a larger-diameter pen and using blank photocopied cheques that had been enlarged and then gradually photocopied in reduced size until he could use a regular cheque book. The signature line was made into a rectangular box with bold outlines for practising and the therapist helped him to use cognitive strategies (based on the CO-OP approach; Rodger and Polatajko, 2017) regarding where to start and finish letters and how to not write over already written letters. Colin also went on to do the crosswords that he enjoyed so much, with the occupational therapist also photocopying these to be larger and helping him develop strategies to keep the letters in the squares.

What is important is that people should not have to wait too long to re-engage in occupations, as our belief is that *doing* will support health and well-being, as well as body function recovery. If an occupational therapist moves away from a focus on occupation to engage in other roles, then the client may miss out on opportunities to re-engage in occupations that are meaningful to him/her, potentially negatively impacting self-efficacy, competence, and life satisfaction and elongating periods of helplessness and dependence.

ACTIVITY

....

Think about the common assessment and intervention tools/techniques or programmes you use or are aware of. Try to map them onto Figure 2.3 as to how close or distant they are to occupational engagement and performance.

LINK BETWEEN OCCUPATION-CENTRED PRACTICE AND PARTICIPATION

There is an increasing recognition within some areas on the importance of participation to health and well-being. Indeed, this is part of what makes up health as described in the International Classification of Functioning, Disability and Health (World Health Organisation, 2001, see Chapter 3).

The focus within much of occupational therapy practice is on enabling the performance of activities, such as helping a child to kick a football. Once the child has developed this skill he/she may have met the immediate goal in relation to occupational therapy. For example, the goal might be *for Johnny to kick a football towards the goal, seven out of 10 tries after three weeks*. However, this is not sufficient for him to participate meaningfully in a football team. A lot of other skills are required to play football: running after the ball without falling over, kicking the ball while running rather than from a stationary position as practiced in therapy, knowing how to be part of a team and knowing the roles of all the player positions etc. The occupation of playing team football and role of team player/ member is much larger than just kicking a football from A to B. Hence, the occupational therapist needs to be cognisant of the many skills required to engage in this occupation and be a fully participating team member.

Coster and Khetani (2008) suggested that participation in life situations can be thought of as a set of organised sequences of activities directed toward a personally or socially meaningful goal. We need to consider how the child will then use his/her skills to participate in the school playground game of football with peers. Bonnard and Anaby (2016) suggested that: "participation can take on both objective (in terms of frequency) and subjective dimensions involving experiences of meaning, belonging, choice, control and the feeling of participation" (p. 188). A focus on participation requires consideration of occupational performance in context. For this it is vital that the occupational therapist understands not only the occupational challenges of a person, but also where and with whom (physical and social environment) the occupational performance is to take place. Working within naturalistic environments helps the occupational therapist to see first-hand the opportunities and challenges associated with participation.

For example, to link occupational performance (kicking a ball from A to B) with participation (playing football) we consider where and when occupation typically takes place. We may be familiar with a football club that is less competitive and more inclusive to children with motor difficulties that we can introduce to the parent. We may spend some time with a coach explaining the child's challenges due to his/her coordination difficulties, and how to enhance his/her performance and acceptance within the team. The focus here is on facilitating real-life participation as a team and club member, enhancing friendships as well as the initial focus of enhancing skill performance regarding kicking goals.

CHAPTER SUMMARY

The unique occupation-centred perspective of occupational therapy is what sets occupational therapists apart from other health care professionals. As occupational therapists, we need to promote the importance of occupation and participation to health and well-being in how we act, what we say and in the services we provide.

Being aware of our reasoning can support the development of occupational therapy practice which is centred on occupation. Top-down reasoning means that your focus throughout the occupational therapy process is on occupation. When we revert to bottom-up and top-to-bottom-up reasoning (which may appear to align more closely with other health care professions' views) it can dilute the effectiveness of occupational therapy.

Understanding the differences between occupation-focused and occupation-based practice is a way of reflecting on occupational therapy services and ensuring our unique perspective is maintained. This is a complex process within many health, social care and education areas where there is often a focus on curing or fixing the underlying impairment in preparation for occupation.

How close or far away occupation is to our practice has implications for the people we work with and for our own professional identity. If we as occupational therapists do not advocate for the importance of occupation to health and well-being, our role can easily turn into one of filling gaps in services and being assistants to other professionals.

Chapter 3, and indeed the remainder of this book, is dedicated to the unpacking of occupation-centred practice and its practical implementation in a variety of settings. Chapter 3 specifically focuses on providing an overview of occupational therapy models, theories and frames of reference. This is to provide you with some background information which will support your reasoning and guide your practice.

REFERENCES

American Occupational Therapy Association (2014) 'Occupational therapy practice framework: Domain and process (3rd edition)'. *American Journal of Occupational Therapy*, *68*, S1–S48.

Bonnard M, Anaby D (2016) 'Enabling participation of students through school-based occupational therapy services: Towards a broader scope of practice'. *British Journal of Occupational Therapy*, *79*(3), 188–192.

Coster WJ, Khetani MA (2008) 'Measuring participation of children with disabilities: Issues and challenge'. *Disability and Rehabilitation*, *30*(8), 639–648.

Dunton WRJ (1919) *Reconstruction therapy*. Philadelphia: WB Saunders. Available at: http://www.dunton.org/archive/biographies/William_Rush_Dunton/Reconstruction_therapy.pdf. Accessed 15/02/18

Estes J, Pierce DE (2012) 'Pediatric therapists' perspectives on occupation-based practice'. *Scandinavian Journal of Occupational Therapy*, *19*(1), 17–25.

Fisher AG (2009) *Occupational therapy intervention process model: A model for planning and implementing top-down, client centred, and occupation-based interventions*. Fort Collins, CO: Three Star Press.

Fisher AG (2013) 'Occupation-centred, occupation-based, occupation-focused: Same, same or different?'. *Scandinavian Journal of Occupational Therapy*, *20*(3), 162–173.

Graham F, Rodger S, Kennedy-Behr A (2017) 'Occupational Performance Coaching (OPC): Enabling caregivers' and children's occupational performance'. In: S Rodger, A Kennedy-Behr, eds, *Occupation-centred practice with children: A practical guide for occupational therapists*. 2nd edn. West Sussex, UK: Wiley-Blackwell, pp. 209–232.

Higgs J, Jones M (2008) 'Clinical decision making and multiple problem spaces'. In: J Higgs, M Jones, S Loftus, N Christensen, eds, *Clinical reasoning in the health professions*. 3rd edn. Edinburgh, UK: Butterworth-Heinemann, pp. 3–17.

Law M, Cooper B, Strong S, Stewart D, Rigby P, Letts L (1996) 'The Person-Environment-Occupational Model: A transactive approach to occupational performance'. *Canadian Journal of Occupational Therapy*, 63(1), 9–23.

Mattingly C, Fleming MH (1994) *Clinical reasoning – Forms of inquiry in a therapeutic practice*. Philadelphia: F.A. Davis.

Novak I, McIntyre S, Morgan C, Campbell L, Dark L, Morton N, Stumbles E, Wilson SA, Goldsmith S (2013) 'A systematic review of interventions for children with cerebral palsy: State of the evidence'. *Developmental Medicine and Child Neurology*, *55*(10), 885–910.

Rodger S, Polatajko HJ (2017) 'Cognitive orientation for daily occupational performance (CO-OP): An occupation-centred intervention'. In: S Rodger, A Kennedy-Behr, eds, *Occupation-centred practice with children: A practical guide for occupational therapists*. 2nd edn. West Sussex, UK: Wiley-Blackwell, pp. 165–188.

Royal College of Occupational Therapists (2015a–last update) *Position statement: Occupation-centred practice*. Available: www.cot.co.uk/position-statements/occupation-centred-practice-august-2015 [March 21, 2017].

Royal College of Occupational Therapists (2015b–last update) *Briefing: Occupation-centred practice*. Available: https://www.rcot.co.uk/practice-resources/learning-zone/cpd-short-courses [December 7, 2017].

Schell BAB, Cervero RM (1993) 'Clinical reasoning in occupational therapy: An integrative review'. *American Journal of Occupational Therapy, 42*, 605–610.

Taylor RR (2008) *The intentional relationship: Occupational therapy and use of self.* Philadelphia: F.A. Davis.

Townsend E, Polatajko HJ, eds (2007) *Enabling occupation II: Advancing an occupational therapy vision for health, well-being and justice through occupation.* Ottawa, ON: CAOT Publications ACE.

Wilcock A (2006) *An occupational perspective on health.* Thorofare, NJ: SLACK Incorporated.

World Federation of Occupational Therapists (2012–last update) *What is occupational therapy?* [Homepage of World Federation of Occupational Therapists], [Online]. Available: www.wfot.org/AboutUs/AboutOccupationalTherapy/WhatisOccupationalTherapy.aspx [October 22, 2016].

World Health Organisation (2001–last update) *International classification of functioning, disability and health.* [Homepage of Author], [Online]. Available: www.who.int/classifications/icf/en/ [October 22, 2016].

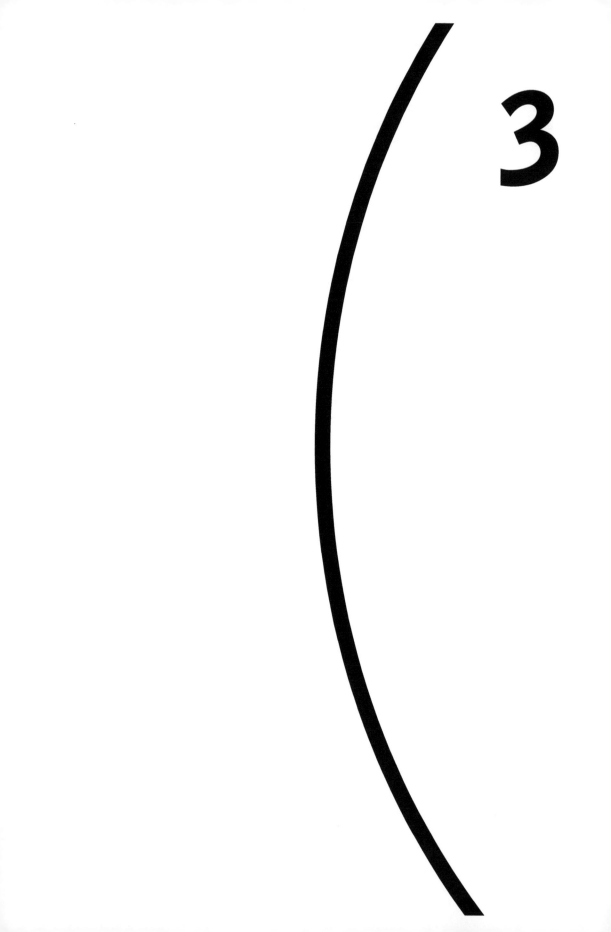

CHAPTER 3
OCCUPATIONAL THERAPY THEORIES AND THE OCCUPATIONAL THERAPY PROCESS

Sylvia Rodger and Karina Dancza

INTENDED CHAPTER OUTCOMES

By the end of this chapter, readers will have an overview of:

- The difference between models, theories and frames of reference
- The International Classification of Functioning, Disability and Health (ICF; World Health Organisation, 2001) as this framework offers a way for occupational therapists to engage with other health and social care professions
- Four key occupational therapy models:
  1 The Person-Environment-Occupation model (PEO; Law, Cooper, Strong, Stewart, Rigby and Letts, 1996)
  2 The Canadian Model of Occupational Performance and Engagement (CMOP-E; Townsend and Polatajko, 2007)
  3 The Model of Human Occupation (MOHO; Kielhofner, 2008)
  4 The Occupational Therapy Intervention Process model (OTIPM; Fisher, 2009)
- The occupational therapy process
- Comparison of occupational therapy models

INTRODUCTION

In this chapter, we provide a brief overview of some key occupational therapy concepts. We define models, theories and frames of reference. The key models we will cover are: (a) the PEO (Law et al., 1996), (b) the CMOP-E (Townsend and Polatajko, 2007), and (c) the MOHO (Kielhofner, 2008) as our experience of education in several countries would suggest that these are the most frequently covered in pre-registration curricula. As well as these occupational therapy specific models, we draw from the ICF (WHO, 2001) as this framework offers a way for occupational therapists to engage with other health and social care professions. We will then describe the occupational therapy process, an iterative sequence of finding out about a client, undertaking assessment, intervening and evaluation of outcomes. Specifically, the Occupational Therapy Intervention Process Model (OTIPM; Fisher, 2009) will be illustrated as this is the occupational therapy process that will be referred to throughout this book.

THEORIES, MODELS, FRAMES OF REFERENCE – KEY DEFINITIONS

Theories explain complex constructs and concepts, their relationships and outcomes (Morse, 1997). Theories, our professional experiences and professional reasoning inform how we operate as occupational therapists (Cohn and Coster, 2014).

Before you began your occupational therapy education, you may have been exposed to a range of formal non-occupational therapy specific theories, such as:

-   Developmental and cognitive theories of psychologists such as Piaget, Erickson and Freud (Crain, 2011)
-   Motor behaviour (Schmidt and Lee, 2005)
-   Social learning theories (Bandura, 1977)
-   Ecological systems theories (such as that by Bronfenbrenner, 1979)

Theories can be broad or overarching (such as theories that help us understand the human need for occupation) or narrower in focus (such as biomechanical theory that tells us about posture and joint movement). Theories help us organise and make sense of our observations and provide insights into our clients' behaviour and performance (Cohn and Coster, 2014).

Professional models delineate the scope of concern or practice of the profession and describe the beliefs and the knowledge held by its members (Cohn and Coster, 2014). The ones that we will address in this chapter include PEO, CMOP-E, MOHO and OTIPM and are broad enough to be used with any occupational therapy client, regardless of his/her age, health condition or the setting in which they are seen. They are not specific enough, however, to guide practice at the level of knowing exactly what to do with a client.

Frames of reference (sometimes called 'practice models') guide practice by outlining key beliefs, assumptions, definitions and concepts, typically within a specific area of practice (Cohn and Coster, 2014). Assessment processes and intervention strategies are typically described that are consistent with the theoretical basis of the frame of reference. One example is the Cognitive Orientation for daily Occupational Performance (CO-OP; Polatajko and Mandich, 2004), which draws from occupational science, behavioural learning theories and dynamic systems theory (Thelen, 1995). These help us to undertake assessments and interventions such as using CO-OP with a child with motor coordination or motor learning difficulties to help him/her ride a bike (Dawson, McEwen and Polatajko, 2017; Polatajko and Mandich, 2004).

In summary, theories, models and frames of reference provide a framework for us to understand the issues or concerns of a client and challenges with which they present. As occupational therapists, we observe and engage with clients using an occupational lens (see Chapter 2), focusing on the occupations our clients prioritise that they need to, want to and must do. Through this lens, theories, models and frames of reference guide us to know how to assess and intervene in a situation.

INTERNATIONAL CLASSIFICATION OF FUNCTIONING, DISABILITY AND HEALTH (ICF)

The ICF (WHO, 2001) has two parts: a classification taxonomy for a range of health conditions and a framework that describes the impact of a health condition on an individual's body structures and function, activities (what they do) and participation (ability to engage in society and their roles). These three aspects are also influenced by personal factors (that are relatively stable and unique to the individual such as ethnicity, gender, socio-economic factors, personality) and environmental factors (family structure, culture, geographic location, institutional context, dwelling) (WHO, 2001). Figure 3.1 illustrates these concepts and their interrelation.

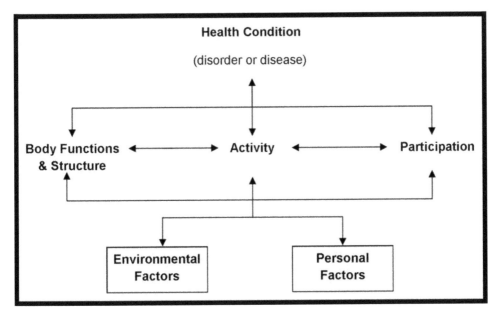

Figure 3.1 The ICF
Reprinted with permission World Health Organisation received 26 October 2016.

As you can see, these concepts are closely related to occupational therapy practice models. When body structure/function issues impact on a person's abilities, these are known as 'impairments'. For example, a stroke (impairment) limits a person's ability to engage in a range of activities depending on the location of the stroke – language, perception, memory, motor functioning needed for dressing, walking, having a conversation. Inability to do these things is known as an 'activity limitation' which also impacts on the person's participation in daily self-care, playing bridge, attending a book club or driving a car. Hence the ICF system can be useful to help categorise the type of difficulties a person might have and the varying contributions of the health condition, the person and the environment to the individual's current activities (limitations) and that impact on his/her participation.

From an occupational therapy perspective, assessment and intervention may occur at the body structure and functions, activity, participation or environment levels. The more occupation-centred the intervention, the more likely the assessment and intervention undertaken will be at the levels of environment, activity and participation. Body structure and function may be a focus, but only if it relates closely to occupation (see Chapter 2 for a discussion of a close focus on occupation). For example, a hand splint provides intervention at the level of body function and structure. Using the splint as one way to assist with handwriting or holding the hand in position for computing or playing bridge, means it is closely related to occupation.

AN OVERVIEW OF FOUR KEY OCCUPATIONAL THERAPY MODELS

In this next section, we will outline four key occupational therapy models. It is recommended that you also refer to other texts and your university learning materials for further detail about these and other models. A useful text to have with you on placement is by Turpin and Iwama (2011), which provides a field guide to a range of occupational therapy models.

The first model we will discuss here is the PEO model developed by Law et al. (1996). It is probably the least complex yet provides an elegant overview of the key constructs underpinning occupational therapy practice.

PERSON–ENVIRONMENT–OCCUPATION MODEL (PEO)

The PEO model draws from environmental behaviour theories, theories of occupation and client- centred practice (Strong, Rigby, Stewart, Law, Letts and Cooper, 1999). The model conceptualises the person, his/her environments and occupations interacting dynamically across the lifespan. The main concepts (P, E, O) are represented by overlapping circles, with occupational performance occurring at the intersection of these circles. The more the circles overlap, the greater the degree of fit and the better the occupational performance is likely to be (Law et al., 1996; Strong et al., 1999). Occupational performance can be enhanced by improving the P-E-O fit. The focus of intervention is to optimise this fit and hence assist the person to optimise their occupational performance.

PERSON

The *person* is the individual who is the centre of the engagement with the occupational therapist. Each client is an individual and the occupational therapist will need to consider:

- His/her age (both developmental and chronological)
- Gender
- The family situation
- Referring challenges and issues
- His/her personality and learning style
- His/her values, strengths and interests
- Presenting conditions (physical, medical or neurological)
- His/her cognitive, sensory, attentional, perceptual abilities
- His/her social and emotional status

Information about these aspects of the person may be obtained through referral sources and information, interviews with the person and relevant others, discussions, observations or other forms of informal and formal assessment.

ENVIRONMENT

Environment in the PEO model refers to the:

- Physical environment (surfaces, size, objects, temperature, other features etc.)
- Social environment – the others (including pets) in the environments where the person functions, such as at home, school, work, neighbourhood/community
- Cultural environment
- Institutional environment, such as workplace with its safety requirements, classrooms with their rules and expectations of students

OCCUPATION

Occupation refers to the self-directed tasks and activities that people engage in over their life course. These clusters of activities and tasks relate to the various roles people assume (Strong et al., 1999). For example, the role of a parent includes activities related to getting themselves and their children washed and dressed, as well as associated activities such as shopping, putting groceries away, caring for pets and caring for one's health care needs (such as taking medications). Within a worker role, activities include going to work at a job each day, completing projects, attending meetings, stacking shelves etc. For children, a role which takes up a considerable amount of time is that of a student. This includes going to school and doing chores like homework tasks, tidying away toys etc. Other occupations might include engaging in leisure interests (such as sports, hobbies, creative pursuits, spiritual activities, relaxation, visiting friends and family etc.). During childhood children learn to look after themselves in terms of bathing, toileting, teeth brushing, dressing etc.

People conduct their daily lives within a range of environments, each with their own supports and challenges, and these vary across the lifespan. Hence it is important for occupational therapists to understand as much as possible about the environments in which occupational challenges occur and what might be the barriers and potential supports that naturally occur in these contexts or could be included to accommodate performance issues.

CHANGE PROCESS

Occupational performance refers to the person's ability to carry out or conduct his/her daily occupations. This sits at the centre of the three overlapping circles in the PEO model. The better the match between the supports and potential for change in the environment, the capacity of the person, and the requirements of the occupation, the better a person's occupational performance will be (Strong et al., 1999). The process of change using the PEO model occurs when the occupational therapist and client work together to address features of each of the P, E, and O that may need altering to optimise the client's occupational performance, the focus of intervention being individualised for each client.

THE CANADIAN MODEL OF OCCUPATIONAL PERFORMANCE AND ENGAGEMENT (CMOP-E)

The CMOP-E (Townsend and Polatajko, 2007/2013) is the second iteration of the Canadian Model of Occupational Performance (CMOP) that was developed in the late 1990s as *Enabling Occupation: An occupational therapy perspective* (Canadian Association of Occupational Therapists, 1997, 2002). The more recent title, *Enabling occupation II,* takes the model to a new level encompassing an occupational vision of health, well-being and justice for all through occupation (Townsend and Polatajko, 2007/2013). What is exceptional about the second iteration is the nation-wide engagement, adoption and writing of various chapters including some 60 Canadian authors. A series of values and beliefs about occupations, the person, the environment, client-centred practice and well-being, health and justice are articulated. This model is grounded in the Canadian health, education and regulatory context and within its socio-culturally diverse population. (Townsend and Polatajko, 2007/2013). As distinct from the initial edition of the model, this version focuses on enabling as a core competency of occupational therapy through the development of the Canadian Model of Client-Centred Enablement (CMCE) and through the Canadian Practice Process Framework (CPPF).

OCCUPATION

The CMOP-E model focuses on occupation as the core domain of concern of occupational therapy with a view that occupation has value as a resource for everyday life. Occupations refer to all manner of human doing or everything people do to occupy themselves categorised as:

- Productivity (contributing to the social economic fabric of communities)
- Self-care (looking after oneself)
- Leisure (enjoying life)

Townsend and Polatajko (2007/2013) outline a taxonomy of occupational performance from actions to tasks to activities to occupations. An occupation being "an activity or set of activities performed with some consistency and regularity, that brings structure and is given value and meaning by individuals and a culture" (Townsend and Polatajko, 2007, p. 19). These are the everyday activities or things that people need to do, have to do and – most importantly – want to do. Occupation in this model is the bridge that connects people to their environment, reinforcing the concept that people act on their environment through doing occupations.

CMOP-E sets out six basic assumptions regarding occupation;

1   Humans need occupations.
2   Occupations affect health and well-being.
3   Occupations organise time and provide structure.
4   Occupations bring meaning to life as ascribed by individuals and cultures.
5   Occupations are idiosyncratic.
6   Occupations have therapeutic potential.

PERSON

In the CMOP-E model, the person (depicted as a triangle in the centre) has three performance components – cognitive, affective and physical – with spirituality as the core (Townsend and Polatajko, 2007/2013). The how, what, where, when and why occupations are engaged in is very much up to the individual person. The *cognitive components* cover elements such as perceptual and intellectual functioning, problem solving, learning style, and reasoning; *affective components* refer to one's emotional and social capacities, personality, self-regulation and self-management; and *physical components* relate to the person's motor control, coordination, sensory capacities, and musculoskeletal and neurological functioning. *Spirituality* sits at the core and refers to the essence of who one is as a human being, epitomising human uniqueness, diversity and personal meaning (Polatajko et al., 2007).

ENVIRONMENT

The person is embedded within the environment, indicating each person's unique environmental context that contains *cultural, institutional, physical and social elements* and that provides occupational opportunities and possibilities (Townsend and Polatajko, 2007/2013). The *physical* environment is both naturally occurring as well as constructed or built. The *social* environment includes the other humans (and pets), whom people interact with in their environment as well as the institutions and culture. The social environment is considered to have micro, meso and macro elements. The micro social environment relates to immediate and personal aspects of daily social interactions, while meso elements refer to social groups existing between the individual and broader social structures. Finally, the macro elements refer to social structures related to policies and regulations of organisations and institutions (Townsend and Polatajko, 2007/2013). The latter may be illustrated by phenomena such as motherhood that are individually, historically, culturally and socially determined and look quite different in various societies. The CMOP-E views culture to be a specific feature of the social environment including values, beliefs, laws, customs, art and creative rituals (Townsend and Polatajko, 2007/2013).

COMPARISONS BETWEEN THE CMOP-E AND ICF

The developers of CMOP-E compared elements of the model with the ICF (WHO, 2001), identifying that body functions and structures as well as personal factors are considered components of the person along with physical, affective, and cognitive functions and structures. Environmental factors in the ICF parallel aspects of the physical, social, cultural and institutional environment. The activity and participation as described in the ICF relate directly to occupational performance and engagement (each person's unique environmental context that contains cultural, institutional, physical and social elements, and that provides occupational opportunities and possibilities (Townsend and Polatajko, 2007). Additionally and uniquely, the developers of CMOP-E propose the use of their model beyond the individual, promoting its use with groups and societies as well promoting occupational justice for all.

CHANGE PROCESS

In the CMOP-E model, change occurs through enabling as described in the Canadian Model of Client-Centred Enablement and through using the Canadian Practice Process Framework. Enabling includes using skills such as adapting, advocating, coaching, collaborating, consulting, coordinating, educating, engaging, designing and specialising (Townsend et al., 2007). The Canadian Practice Process Framework offers an occupational therapy process to support therapists in articulating the model in practice.

MODEL OF HUMAN OCCUPATION (MOHO)

The development of the MOHO in the late 1970s coincided with the renaissance of occupation within the occupational therapy profession (Taylor, 2017). In the preceding period since the 1940s, most occupational therapists were focusing on body structures and function and impairment reduction (Forsyth et al., 2014). The MOHO shifted the focus of occupational therapists to generating an understanding of how a person engages in occupation. MOHO proposes that inner capacities, motives and patterns of performance are maintained and changed through occupational engagement. Clients' abilities, routines, thoughts and feelings are shaped via their engagement in occupations (Forsyth et al., 2014). MOHO utilises concepts of the person, the environment, occupational participation, performance and skill (Forsyth et al., 2014).

PERSON

Specific concepts in the MOHO model relate to *the person*. These intrinsic characteristics are volition, habituation and performance capacity (Forsyth et al., 2014).

Volition refers to motivation toward and choice of activities. Volition consists of interests, sense of abilities (personal causation) and values. *Interests* arise from the experience, pleasure and satisfaction derived from doing occupations. *Personal causation* conveys a person's capacity and effectiveness related to doing everyday activities. *Values* refer to beliefs and commitments about what is good, right and important for a person to do (Taylor, 2017).

Habituation refers to the way in which people organise actions into patterns and routines. These habits are learned ways of doing that become automatic. *Roles* provide an identity and sense of obligation and a way of behaving. Roles become internalised over time (Taylor, 2017).

Finally, *performance capacity* refers to underlying mental and physical abilities and their use in performance. This capacity is influenced by a range of body structures and functions (cognition, memory, musculoskeletal, neurological, cardio respiratory status). A person's experiences of performance are as important as a person's capacities (Taylor, 2017).

ENVIRONMENT

MOHO (Forsyth et al., 2014) also contains concepts concerning the *environment*. Occupation results from an interaction of the intrinsic characteristics of the person and the environment (physical and social). In MOHO terms, the environment refers to the spaces humans occupy, the objects they use and the people in the context. The environment offers potential opportunities and challenges for occupational performance and these interact with the person's intrinsic characteristics (volition, habituation and performance capacity). The environment also includes the occupational opportunities which are available, expected, and required of people in given contexts, or social groups, and the macro cultural, political and economic climate (Taylor, 2017).

OCCUPATION

In terms of *occupation*, MOHO contains three concepts: occupational participation, performance and skill (Forsyth et al., 2014). Occupational participation refers to engaging in work, play and self-care activities that are part of one's sociocultural context and are necessary and/or desired. Occupational performance refers to the doing of tasks related to participation in major life areas. Skills refer to the actions that comprise the occupational performance.

CHANGE PROCESS

According to Kielhofner (2008), what people engage in doing creates their individual occupational identity. This doing is referred to as 'occupational competence'. Both occupational identity and competence are outcomes of the engagement of people in occupations. What a client does, thinks or feels impacts on the process of therapeutic change. Most important in therapy are concepts of volition, habituation, performance capacity and the environment. When using MOHO, there are six key steps in therapeutic reasoning (Forsyth et al., 2014) that therapists use to guide the process of change. These are outlined in Table 3.1.

Table 3.1 Six key steps in MOHO-based therapeutic reasoning

MOHO Reasoning Steps	Comments
Generating questions	MOHO practitioners consider a person's thoughts and feelings re. causation, values and interests.
Gathering information	Many structured assessments based on MOHO constructs have been developed, such as the Assessment of Motor and Process Skills (AMPS), Pediatric Interest Profiles (PIP) and School Setting Interview (SSI).
Creating a theory-based understanding of the person	A conceptualisation of the person's circumstances is created using MOHO constructs such as volition, habits and performance capacity.
Generating therapy goals and strategies	Therapy goals are created as well as the strategies required to support change. Goals are identified with the person that involve occupational engagement in the person's typical environment.
Implementing and monitoring therapy	These occur iteratively through the person's occupational engagement and therapist's use of a range of strategies including providing feedback, advising, negotiating, structuring choice, coaching, encouraging and providing physical support.
Collecting information to assess outcomes	MOHO is one of the few occupational therapy models for which there has been significant investment by researchers in the development of MOHO-based evaluation measures that are conceptually consistent with key MOHO concepts (e.g., Volition Questionnaire).

Created by Sylvia Rodger, November 2016, based on Kielhofner et al. (2009, pp. 450–455).

THE OCCUPATIONAL THERAPY INTERVENTION PROCESS MODEL (OTIPM)

To structure occupational therapy involvement and remain focused on the unique contributions of the occupational therapist, it is important to work through a specific process. This occupational therapy process provides a series of steps to follow, and brings together our thinking about theories, practice models, frame(s) of reference and specific approaches.

This chapter, and indeed this book, will utilise the Occupational Therapy Intervention Process Model (OTIPM; Fisher, 2009, p. 16, updated by Fisher, 2013, p. 7). This model outlines the process of occupational therapy intervention through three phases of evaluation and goal setting, intervention and re-evaluation. It is illustrated in Figure 3.2.

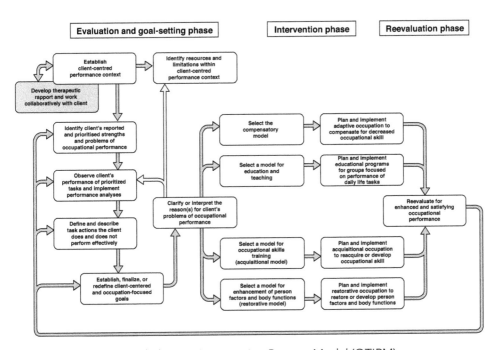

Figure 3.2 Occupational Therapy Intervention Process Model (OTIPM)

Adapted from: Fisher (2009). Available: www.innovativeotsolutions.com/content/wp-content/uploads/2014/01/English-OTIPM-handout.pdf. Reprinted with permission.

Fisher (2009) holds many of the beliefs outlined in the CMOP-E. Specifically, she describes (a) the uniqueness of the individual and his/her sense of meaning and purpose for doing, (b) a client's engagement in occupation as the central focus of the profession, (c) therapeutic use of occupation as the profession's primary 'means' and (d) clients' engagement in meaningful occupation as the primary 'end'. The OTIPM is used in conjunction with client-centred, top-down, occupation-based approach to assessment and intervention. It aims to provide a structure to guide professional reasoning.

OCCUPATION

In the OTIPM, Fisher (2009) outlines key constructs such as 'occupation' from the perspective of actions in which people engage. The person's *engagement in the process of doing* is critical to the construct of occupation. These occupations take place *within a space, over a period and within the context of a person's life roles* such as being a parent or school student. For example, the occupational therapist might observe a series of actions undertaken by a parent in the task of getting a child ready for school. These actions may involve making the child's lunch, getting the child out of bed, supervising dressing in uniform, putting things out for breakfast, supervising teeth cleaning and ensuring the child leaves in time to catch the bus.

Fisher (2009) focuses on the *meaning or significance of occupations* for people. Occupations can have both meaning and purpose. For example, a retiree may engage in volunteering at a local school reading to children or listening to them read. This occupation of

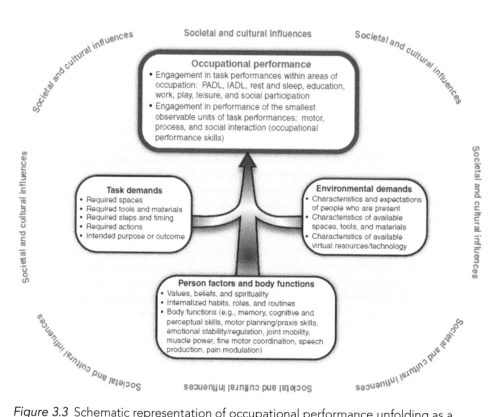

Figure 3.3 Schematic representation of occupational performance unfolding as a transaction among person factors and body functions, task demands, environmental demands and societal and cultural influences

Adapted from Fisher (2009). Available: www.innovativeotsolutions.com/content/wp-content/uploads/2014/01/English-OTIPM-handout.pdf. Reprinted with permission.

volunteering may have meaning for the retiree as she feels that she can give back to the community now that she has more time. It may also have purpose for her as her grandchild attends that school and this enables her to spend time with him.

Fisher (2009) outlines how occupational performance (the focus of the model) "unfolds as a transaction between the person and the environment as he/she enacts a task" (p. 44). The constructs of environment, person and occupational performance are illustrated in the schematic representation which accompanies the OTIPM process (Figure 3.3).

ENVIRONMENT

In Figure 3.3 the environment is considered as the environmental demands relating to where the occupational performance takes place. This includes the characteristics and expectations of the people present (which could be considered aligned with the social context in CMOP-E and PEO); the characteristics of the available spaces, tools and materials (the physical environment); and the characteristics of the available virtual resources and technology. In the OTIPM process, the term 'performance context' is used and this most closely parallels the term 'environment' used in other models. Performance context refers to where the person engages in their occupations.

Where possible the therapist is guided to observe performance in context and to identify the resources and limitations within the person's context. This is akin to understanding how the context (environment) supports or hinders the person's performance and guides the therapist to consider how modifications to the environment might assist the person to perform more optimally. The *client-centred performance context* comprises a range of dimensions: environmental, role, motivational, task, cultural, social, societal, body function, temporal and finally adaptational (Fisher, 2009, p. 44). Dimensions such as environmental, cultural, social, societal and temporal are dimensions that are seen in the environment component of other models discussed.

PERSON

The occupational therapist is guided to "establish client centred performance context" which is the first step depicted in the flow diagram (Figure 3.2) (Fisher, 2009, p. 16). While the term 'person' is not used specifically, there is reference throughout the process to the client and much focus is placed on the occupational therapist developing therapeutic rapport and collaborative relationships with the client (person) and significant others. In terms of the client, dimensions of interest in this model are their roles, motivations, body function and adaptation, as shown in Figure 3.3.

Rather than focusing on aspects of the client in Figure 3.3 articulated in other models, the flow diagram of the OTIPM (Figure 3.2) shows how the OTIPM moves directly to having the occupational therapist gather information about the client's strengths and problems from his/her perspective in relation to *occupational performance* and then observing the person doing the task (i.e., task performance). This requires the occupational therapist to engage in performance analysis to enable him/her to identify the actions the client can do competently and those that are problematic. The analysis occurs from the perspective of the motor, process and social interaction performance skills that the client requires to undertake the occupational performance. This process is outlined in detail in Chapter 4.

CHANGE PROCESS

Change is mapped by the occupational therapist using the OTIPM flow diagram (Figure 3.2) to step through developing an understanding of the client and his/her performance context, goal prioritisation, observation and assessment, choice of relevant intervention approaches, and finally re-evaluation.

During the intervention phase of the OTIPM (Figure 3.2), the occupational therapist's task is to select an intervention model or approach to support change. The approaches are described as compensatory, education and training, occupational skill development or training (acquisition) or enhancement of person factors and body functions (restorative). Whilst not mutually exclusive (one intervention may use a combination of approaches), the focus of each is:

- **Adaptive approaches** focus on the use of technology, compensatory techniques or modifications of the task or the physical and social environment to assist a person to manage his/her occupational performance.
- **Educational interventions** provide information to groups of people related to strategies they can use to enhance daily life and occupational performance.

- **Acquisitional approaches** focus on assisting clients to develop or acquire new or lost skills to enable the goal-directed actions needed for occupational performance.
- **Restorative approaches** focus on remediating underlying impairments, development or maintenance of person factors and body functions underlying occupational performance. The OTIPM specifies that any restorative approaches must be undertaken within occupations, such as going swimming or horse-riding to improve core strength, balance or self-esteem.

COMPARING THE MODELS

When making decisions about what over-arching model to use, it is important to be able to compare the models and understand the focus of each. While the key constructs – person, environment and occupation or occupational performance – are similar, there are subtle differences in the definitions and focus of each model. For example, in MOHO occupational performance is an outcome of the interaction between person and environment, rather than there being a focus on occupation; whereas in PEO, CMOP-E and OTIPM, occupation features as a key component. The following Figures (3.4, 3.5, 3.6 and 3.7) demonstrate the differences between models regarding how each of the constructs of person, environment and occupation, as well as the process of change is articulated in each model.

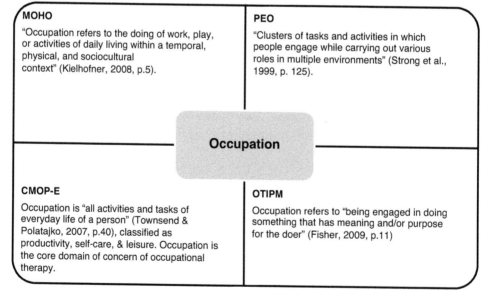

Figure 3.4 Overview of *Occupation* as described by four models

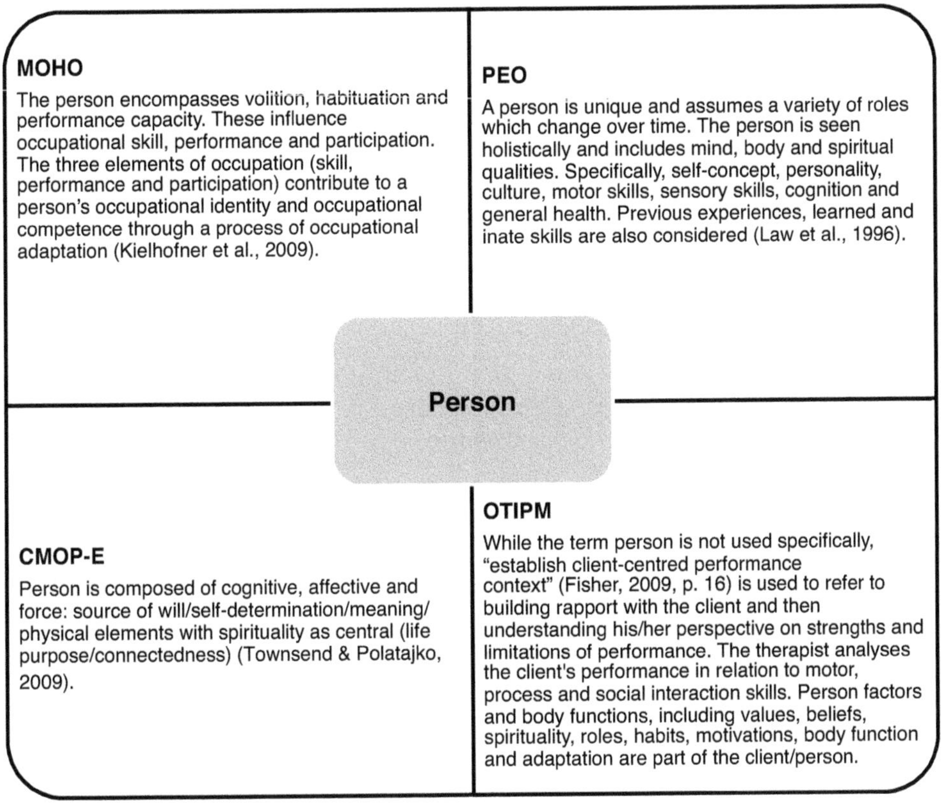

MOHO

The person encompasses volition, habituation and performance capacity. These influence occupational skill, performance and participation. The three elements of occupation (skill, performance and participation) contribute to a person's occupational identity and occupational competence through a process of occupational adaptation (Kielhofner et al., 2009).

PEO

A person is unique and assumes a variety of roles which change over time. The person is seen holistically and includes mind, body and spiritual qualities. Specifically, self-concept, personality, culture, motor skills, sensory skills, cognition and general health. Previous experiences, learned and inate skills are also considered (Law et al., 1996).

Person

CMOP-E

Person is composed of cognitive, affective and force: source of will/self-determination/meaning/physical elements with spirituality as central (life purpose/connectedness) (Townsend & Polatajko, 2009).

OTIPM

While the term person is not used specifically, "establish client-centred performance context" (Fisher, 2009, p. 16) is used to refer to building rapport with the client and then understanding his/her perspective on strengths and limitations of performance. The therapist analyses the client's performance in relation to motor, process and social interaction skills. Person factors and body functions, including values, beliefs, spirituality, roles, habits, motivations, body function and adaptation are part of the client/person.

Figure 3.5 Overview of the *Person* as described by four models

MOHO

The environment refers to the physical, social, cultural, economic and political features of the person's context that influence his/her motivation, organisation and occupational performance (Kielhofner et al., 2009).

PEO

"Broadly includes the cultural, institutions, physical and social factors influencing occupation performance" (Strong et al., 1999, p. 125).

Environment

CMOP-E

Each person has a unique environmental context that contains cultural, institutional, physical and social elements and that provides occupational opportunities and possibilities (Townsend & Polatajko, 2007).

OTIPM

The term *performance context* rather than environment is used. Performance context refers to where the person engages in their occupations. Environmental, cultural, social, societal, and temporal dimensions are described as theoretical assumptions of the model (Fisher, 2009).

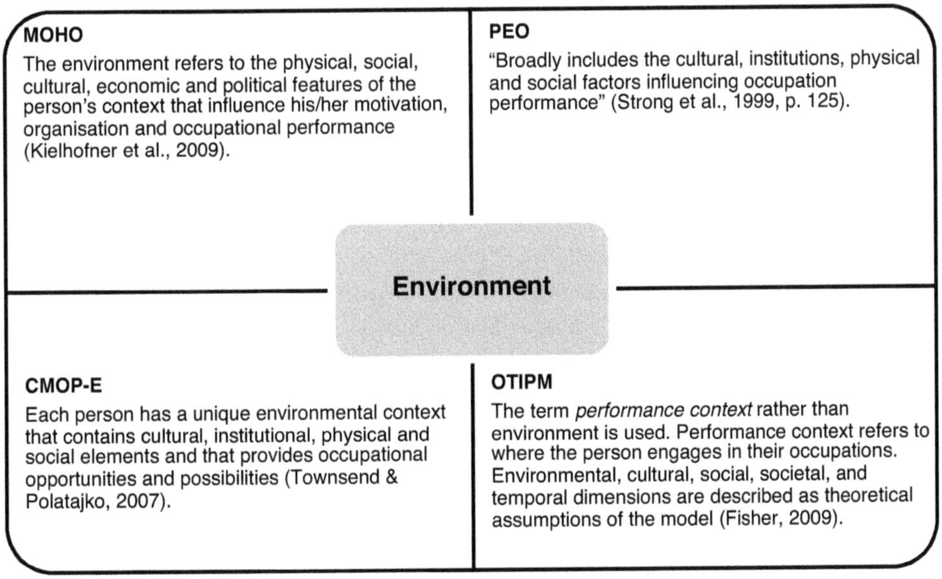

Figure 3.6 Overview of the *Environment* as described by four models

MOHO	PEO
By enhancing a person's volition, habits and capacity and/or by changing elements of the environment, the therapist works to enable the person to realise their values and interests through occupation. Intervention within MOHO to improve occupational performance is designed to affect change in volition, habituation or performance capacity. MOHO (Kielhofner, 2008, p. 29) argues that changes in occupational performance occur as a result of changes in any or all of these elements; "ordinarily, volition, habituation, and performance capacity change in concert" (Kielhofner, 2008, p. 126).	Occupational performance can be enhanced by improving the P-E-O fit. The focus of intervention is on optimising this fit (Law et al., 1996). Change occurs via improving P-E-O fit or overlap.

Process of Change

CMOP-E	OTIPM
Change occurs through enabling as described in the The Canadian Model of Client-Centred Enablement (CMCE) and through using the Canadian Practice Process Framework (CPPF). Enabling includes a range of skills such as adapting, advocating, coaching, collaborating, consulting, coordinating, educating, engaging, designing, and specialising (Townsend & Polatajko, 2007/2013) utilised by the therapist to facilitate change.	Intervention can involve addressing disruptions in any of the 10 interrelated dimensions of the client-centred performance context (Fisher, 2009, p. 44). Embedded within the OTIPM is a compensatory model of intervention. The OTIPM also offers occupational therapists the option of using restorative, acquisitional or educative models of intervention which are explained in other literature. However by using the OTIPM reasoning process, compensatory, educative, acquisitional or restorative models of intervention must be implemented in a manner which is "truly top-down, client-centred, and occupation-based" (Fisher, 2009, p. 43).

Figure 3.7 Overview of the *Process of Change* as described by four models

CHAPTER SUMMARY

In this chapter, we have provided a definition of theories, models and frames of reference. We have then provided a brief overview of the ICF and four occupational therapy models – PEO, CMOP-E, MOHO, and OTIPM. These occupational therapy models provide information about the domain of concern of occupational therapy and we outlined their perspectives regarding constructs of person, environment and occupation, as well as the process of change. We described how these models relate to the ICF as a more generic view of how health conditions impact on a person's activities and participation. We then introduced how the OTIPM provides an intervention process for occupational therapists to follow in engaging with individual clients. We compared all four models in terms of their key constructs to highlight their similarities and differences. It is anticipated that you may need to come back regularly to this chapter to consolidate key concepts and elements of the intervention process, while reading and working through other chapters in this book.

REFERENCES

Bandura A (1977) 'Self-efficacy: Toward a unifying theory of behavioural change'. *Psychological Review, 84*(2), 191–215.

Bronfenbrenner U (1979) *The ecology of human development: Experiments by nature and design.* Cambridge, MA: Harvard University Press.

Canadian Association of Occupational Therapists (1997) *Enabling occupation: An occupational therapy perspective.* Ottawa, ON: CAOT Publications ACE.

Canadian Association of Occupational Therapists (2002) *Enabling occupation: An occupational therapy perspective.* Revised edn. Ottawa, ON: CAOT Publications ACE.

Crain W (2011) *Theories of development: Concepts and applications.* 6th edn. Abingdon, Oxon: Routledge.

Cohn ES, Coster WJ (2014) 'Unpacking our theoretical reasoning: theory and practice in occupational therapy'. In: BAB Schell, G Gillen, ME Scaffa, eds, *Willard & Spackman's occupational therapy.* 12th edn. Philadelphia, PA: Lippincott Williams & Wilkins, pp. 478–493.

Dawson D, McEwen S, Polatajko HJ, eds (2017) *The CO-OP approach: Enabling participation across the lifespan.* Bethesda, MD: American Occupational Therapy Association Press.

Fisher AG (2009) *Occupational therapy intervention process model: A model for planning and implementing top-down, client centred, and occupation-based interventions.* Fort Collins, CO: Three Star Press.

Fisher AG (2013) 'Occupation-centred, occupation-based, occupation-focused: Same, same or different?'. *Scandinavian Journal of Occupational Therapy, 20*(3), 162–173.

Forsyth K, Taylor RR, Kramer JM, Prior S, Richie L, Whitehead J, Owen C and Melton J (2014) 'The model of human occupation'. In: BAB Schell, G Gillen, ME Scaffa, eds, *Willard & Spackman's occupational therapy.* 12th edn. Philadelphia, PA: Lippincott Williams & Wilkins, pp. 505–526.

Kielhofner G (2008) *A model of human occupation: Theory and application.* 4th edn. Baltimore, MD: Lippincott Williams & Wilkins.

Kielhofner G, Forsyth K, Kramer JM, Melton J, Dobson E (2009) 'The model of human occupation'. In: EB Crepeau, ES Cohn, BA Boyt Schell, eds, *Willard &*

Spackman's occupational therapy. 11th edn. Baltimore, MD: Lippincott Williams & Wilkins, pp. 444–461.

Law M, Cooper B, Strong S, Stewart D, Rigby P, Letts L (1996) 'The Person-Environment-Occupational Model: A transactive approach to occupational performance'. *Canadian Journal of Occupational Therapy*, 63(1), 9–23.

Morse JM (1997) 'Considering theory derived from qualitative research'. In: JM Morse, ed, *Completing a qualitative project: Details and dialogues*. Thousand Oaks, CA: Sage Publications, pp. 163–188.

Polatajko HJ, Mandich A (2004) *Enabling occupation in children: The cognitive orientation to daily occupational performance (CO-OP) approach*. Ottawa, ON: CAOT Publications ACE.

Polatajko HJ, Molke D, Baptiste S, Doble S, Santha JC, Kirsh B, Beagan BL, Kumas-Tan Z, Iwama M, Laliberte Rudman D, Thibeault R and Stadnyk R. (2007) 'Occupational science imperatives for occupational therapy'. In: E Townsend, HJ Polatajko, eds, *Enabling occupation II: Advancing an occupational therapy vision for health, well-being and justice through occupation*. Ottawa, ON: CAOT Publications ACE, pp. 63–82.

Schmidt RA, Lee TD (2005) *Motor control and learning: A behavioural emphasis*. 4th edn. Champaign, IL: Human Kinetics.

Strong S, Rigby P, Stewart D, Law M, Letts L, Cooper B (1999) 'Application of the Person-Environment-Occupation Model: A practical tool'. *Canadian Journal of Occupational Therapy*, 66(3), 122–133.

Taylor R (2017) *Kielhofner's model of human occupation: Theory and application*. 5th edn. Philadelphia, PA: Lippincott Williams and Wilkins.

Thelen E (1995) 'Motor development: A new synthesis'. *American Psychologist*, 50(2), 79–95.

Townsend E, Polatajko HJ, eds (2007/2013) *Enabling occupation II: Advancing an occupational therapy vision for health, well-being and justice through occupation*. Ottawa, ON: CAOT Publications ACE.

Turpin M, Iwama MK (2011) *Using occupational therapy models in practice: A field guide*. London, UK: Churchill Livingstone Elsevier.

World Health Organisation (2001–last update) *International classification of functioning, disability and health*. [Homepage of Author], [Online]. Available: www.who.int/classifications/icf/en/ [October 22, 2016].

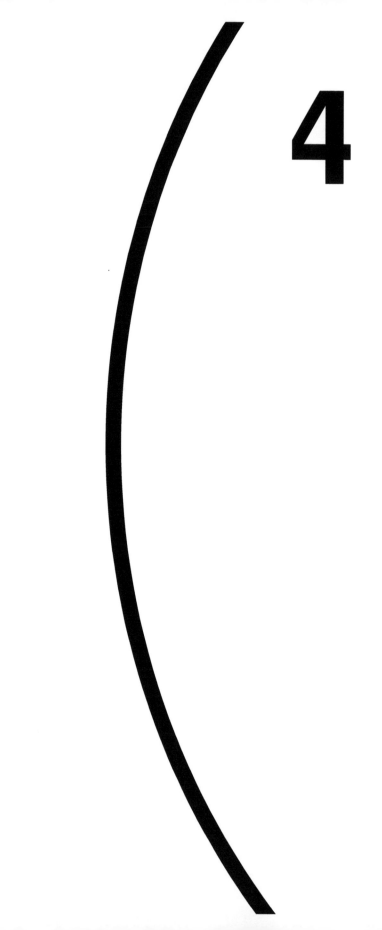

4

CHAPTER 4

KEY TOOLS OF THE OCCUPATIONAL THERAPIST: OCCUPATIONAL PROFILING, ACTIVITY ANALYSIS AND OCCUPATIONAL PERFORMANCE ANALYSIS

Karina Dancza, Jeannette Head and Sue Mesa

INTENDED CHAPTER OUTCOMES

By the end of this chapter, readers will have an overview of:

- Occupational profiling and how it can be used to guide a client-centred occupational therapy process
- The use of activity analysis to support reasoning and intervention planning
- Using observation and occupational performance analysis as key assessment tools
- Practical examples and templates which could be used in practice settings

INTRODUCTION

For occupational therapists, occupation and its relationship to health and well-being is our unique perspective. What is different about an occupational therapy assessment and that of other professionals is that we observe and analyse what people do, the quality of the smallest units of performance (i.e. the performance skills) as they unfold over time (Chard and Mesa, 2017). Therefore, we need tools to help understand how someone does his/her occupations, so that we can use this knowledge to inform our intervention plans and support participation.

This chapter introduces you to three core tools of occupational therapy: occupational profiling, activity analysis and occupational performance analysis. For coherence and clarity as you learn the occupational therapy process, we will use these tools and associated templates as examples in Part II of this book. This does not, however, preclude you from using other assessments. You may find that once you are familiar with the occupational therapy process and understand how to use these tools to support your decision making, you can critically compare and select the most appropriate tools. Our intention here is to provide you with one way as a starting point in your learning.

IS IT AN OCCUPATION, ACTIVITY OR TASK?

Occupations are complex and so too is the terminology surrounding them. Some authors use terms to describe subtly different things, whilst others do not recognise a difference (Chard and Mesa, 2017; Christiansen and Townsend, 2014; Mackenzie and O'Toole, 2011; Pierce, 2003). Consider the terms 'occupation', 'activity' and 'task' for one such illustration.

'Activity' or 'task' describes a *general* way in which something is done (Pierce, 2003). Considering the finest detail of the way in which something is typically done is what happens when we undertake an activity or task analysis (this will be explored further within this chapter). Chard and Mesa (2017) suggest that 'activity' and 'task' mean the same thing, despite some authors separating out these two terms. For clarity, in this chapter and throughout this book these terms will be used to mean the same thing.

There is, however, a difference between the words 'activity' and 'occupation'. Chard and Mesa (2017, p. 212) offer a suggestion for differentiating between these two terms: "activity is a shared concept about 'what' is done. It becomes an occupation when a person does the occupation (it is observable) and it has individual meaning and purpose to the person." This is similar to how the World Federation of Occupational Therapists (2012) defines *occupation*. They describe it as "The everyday activities that people do as individuals, in families and with communities to occupy time and bring meaning and purpose to life. Occupations include things people need to, want to and are expected to do." A summary of activity, task and occupation terms and definitions are presented in Table 4.1.

Table 4.1 Summary of activity, task and occupation terms

Activity or Task	A shared concept about *what* is done
Occupation	When a person occupies his/her time doing something (it is observable) and it has meaning and purpose

KEY TOOLS OF THE OCCUPATIONAL THERAPIST

Occupational profiling, *activity analysis* and *occupational performance analysis* comprise the 'engine house' of occupational therapy. They are our primary tools within an occupation-centred approach.

OCCUPATIONAL PROFILING

An *occupational profile* (American Occupational Therapy Association, 2014) of our client develops as we gather information about the occupational strengths, needs, wishes and circumstances of the person (Fisher, 2009). This is often undertaken via interview with the person, his/her family and significant others, along with a review of documentation such as case notes, medical records and previous reports. In the Occupational Therapy Intervention Process Model (OTIPM; Fisher, 2009), this would be termed 'establishing the client-centred performance context' (see Chapter 6 for details).

From this initial information gathering, we collaboratively determine with the person (and relevant others) the occupations he/she would like to prioritise. The interview process assists us in developing rapport with the person and his/her significant others. It is important to spend time developing rapport to ensure the prioritisation process is successful in identifying which occupations are relevant and meaningful to the person as this will guide the remainder of our occupational therapy involvement (Chard and Mesa, 2017).

The creation of an occupational profile is the starting point for your occupational therapy process. It enables you to begin to understand your clients as occupational beings and it may also help your clients consider their occupations as important parts of their own health and well-being. You may also discuss with your clients what they want to, need to, or are expected to do and how they see the balance between self-care, productive and leisure roles, including roles which they may like in the future.

When you are clear about the priority occupation(s) you and your client will focus on during your occupational therapy involvement, you need to ensure you have a thorough understanding of the demands of those occupations. This is where you can use activity analysis.

ACTIVITY ANALYSIS

An *activity analysis* (or some might call it 'task analysis') involves breaking down an activity into the components that influence how it is *chosen*, *organised* and *carried out* within the *environment* in which it might be typically performed (Creek, 2010). We use activity analysis to identify the inherent demands, requirements and meanings of activities to determine what is 'fixed' (i.e. can't be changed) and what is 'flexible' (i.e. could be changed) (Creek, 2010; Mackenzie and O'Toole, 2011). This helps us not only in thinking about intervention potential, but it also can assist us in considering potential areas of risk which we need to be aware of as we move through the occupational therapy process.

With appropriate research, you can gain an understanding of an activity even if you have limited experience of it. For example, you may have no experience of indoor rock climbing, so you look up how to do it by viewing clips on the internet or speaking with an instructor at the local leisure centre. Through this research, you can gain a general appreciation of peoples' participation in indoor rock climbing.

To gain a detailed understanding, we need to break down the activity into the smallest observable parts. To achieve this, we need to consider the *steps* and *actions* involved in how a *human* would typically undertake the activity. A *step* is a structured series of actions with a recognisable end product (Chard and Mesa, 2017). An *action* is the doing of something, not what is done; actions can be described using 'doing' words, such as grasp*ing*, reach*ing* or ask*ing*. These are the smallest observable units of participation (Chard and Mesa, 2017). An example of breaking down the activity of brushing your teeth into steps and actions is illustrated in Table 4.2.

There are many ways of carrying out an activity analysis. We will describe one way to capture these considerations which we have modified from Head, Gray and Dancza (2014). This is illustrated in Table 4.3 and downloadable from www.routledge.com/9781138238480. The activity analysis template is divided into four sections:

1   The potential purpose of the activity
2   The characteristics of the contexts where the activity could be done
3   A detailed breakdown of the activity into steps and actions
4   Consideration of how a person's body functions and structures (e.g. things *inside* the person such as strength, posture, memory) combine to enable the activity to take place

Table 4.2 Steps and actions of brushing teeth

Step	Action
Collect toothbrush and toothpaste.	Walking to the cupboard Grasping and opening cupboard door Reaching for and grasping toothbrush and toothpaste
Put toothpaste onto toothbrush.	Grasping and manipulating toothpaste cap to open it Squeezing toothpaste onto toothbrush Manipulating toothpaste cap closed
Brush teeth.	Grasping toothbrush Moving the toothbrush around in the mouth
Rinse toothbrush.	Reaching for, grasping and turning on the tap Rinsing toothbrush and placing it back in the cupboard
Rinse mouth.	Reaching for, grasping and lifting cup, moving cup under tap to fill Lifting cup to mouth to sip, moving water around mouth and spitting out

Table 4.3 Activity analysis template

Name of activity _____

Section 1: Potential purpose

Why might a person do this activity?

Section 2: Potential contexts

Required physical space

Where is the activity typically done? Describe the physical environment such as size of space, physical arrangement of furniture, accessibility, surfaces (flooring, walls), lighting (natural/artificial), temperature, noise, humidity and ventilation.

Required objects

What tools, materials or equipment are required? Describe the properties of each such as type, size, shape, weight, texture and position of use.

Required social context

Can the activity be done by one person or does it need more than one person? Does the activity require social interactions or forming relationships? Does the activity require the sharing of personal information such as feelings, life experiences, thoughts, ideas, values, or beliefs? Does the activity require learning from others, cooperation, or competition with others? What are the social and cultural expectations, rules and norms?

Required temporal context

When does the activity take place and how frequently – daily, weekly, monthly, by necessity, by choice, at a specific time of day, week, month or year? Does the activity typically happen before or after another activity? How long does the activity take?

Section 3: Steps and actions

Required sequence

Steps	Actions
A step is a stage in the activity. Steps comprise of series of actions with a recognisable output.	*An action is the smallest observable unit of performance (do<u>ing</u> words).*
List in order the steps typically required to complete each task. Consider: – Is the order fixed or flexible? – How long does each step take? – What is the typical speed of performance?	*List in order the actions typically required to complete each step.*

(Continued)

Table 4.3 (Continued)

Section 4: Body functions and structures

What are the essential body functions and structures associated with the steps of the activity?

You may need to consider this for individual steps and associated actions. There are multiple body functions and structures required when doing each step. Think about the primary ones which might cause an issue if the person had difficulties associated with it when doing a step. You could revisit this thinking about diagnoses or conditions (e.g. dementia, cerebral palsy, limb amputation etc.). A list of body functions, which is organised according to the classifications of the ICF, follows to help you think about the many factors within the person which could impact on performance. For fuller descriptions of body functions, please refer to WHO (2001).

Body functions	Body function prompts	Body function definitions
Mental functions (including affective, cognitive and perceptual)	Consciousness	Level of consciousness, arousal
	Orientation	To person, place, time, self and others
	Intellectual	Retardation, dementia
	Energy and drive	Motivation, impulse control, interests, values
	Sleep	Quality, quantity, sleep patterns
	Attention	Sustained and divided
	Memory	Retrospective, prospective
	Emotion	Appropriate range and regulation of emotions, self-control
	Perception	Visuospatial, body schema, sensory interpretation
	Higher cognitive functions	Executive functions of judgement, concept formation, time management, problem solving, decision making
	Psychomotor functions	Experience of self, regulation of motor response to psychological events, motor planning
	Language functions	Receive and express self through spoken/ written/sign language
	Calculation functions	Ability to calculate (add and subtract etc.)
Sensory functions and pain	Seeing	Visual acuity, visual field
	Hearing	Responding to sounds, pitch and volume
	Vestibular	Balance
	Gustatory	Taste, including smell

Table 4.3 (Continued)

Body functions	Body function prompts	Body function definitions
Sensory functions and pain (continued)	Touch	Sensitivity to touch, ability to discriminate
	Proprioceptive	Kinaesthesia, joint position sense
	Pain	Pain sensation – dull/stabbing/ache
Voice and speech functions	Voice	Articulate and produce sounds, words and communication
Cardiovascular, haematological, immunological and respiratory functions	Heart	Pulse rate, physical endurance, stamina, fatigue
	Blood pressure	Hypotension, hypertension, postural hypotension
	Haematological	Blood
	Immune response	Allergies, hypersensitivity
	Respiration	Breathing, rate, rhythm, depth
Digestive, metabolic and endocrine systems functions	Digestive/ defecation	Food intake/output
	Weight maintenance	Diet, obesity
	Endocrine glands	Hormonal changes
Genitourinary and reproductive functions	Urination	Fluid intake/output, micturition
	Sexual functions	Libido, pregnancy, birth
Neuromuscular and movement-related functions	Mobility of joints	Range of motion, postural alignment, joint stability/mobility
	Muscle power	Strength, endurance
	Muscle tone	Degree of tone, spasticity, flaccidity
	Movement functions	Hand–eye and foot coordination, bilateral integration, walking patterns and gait
	Involuntary movements	Motor reflexes, righting reactions, tics, tremors, motor perseveration
Skin and related functions	Skin	Presence/absence of wounds, cuts, abrasions; healing
	Hair and nail	Protective, appearance

A cautionary note – *steps and actions are visible* during an observation. *Body functions and structures underpin actions, but cannot be directly observed during activity* as these happen within the body. For example, it might be assumed that when you see someone start to find a cup, pause, then start to fill the kettle and never return to searching for the cup, that you are observing poor memory. Or when you see someone drop a saucepan, you are observing reduced strength. In these cases, you are *assuming* the cause of the person's challenges (memory or strength). If you jump to these conclusions too early, you are in danger of missing other factors which may also have contributed (e.g. distraction within the room or the slippery nature of an object). Therefore, within your activity analysis, ensure you note what is *observable* (steps and actions) and then consider the *multiple* body functions and structures required for each step (see Section 4 in Table 4.3).

An example of a completed activity analysis is shown in Table 4.4. This illustrates how activity analysis can be used to consider making beans on toast with cheese. Whilst initially completing the template may be an arduous task, the detail generated and understanding of the complexity of the occupation gained are invaluable. Through this process of analysing activities, the intervention potential for grading and adaptation of steps and actions is highlighted.

Table 4.4 Activity analysis example

Name of activity: Making lunch of beans on toast with cheese

Section 1: Potential purpose

- To cook lunch for yourself to demonstrate your independence
- To gain nutrition
- Because you enjoy cooking

Section 2: Potential contexts

Required physical space
A kitchen with space to walk in, places to put a plate and other objects needed. A bench to put things on. Lighting to see the required objects and a comfortable temperature, noise, humidity. The floor is not too slippery or cluttered so a person can stand or sit on a stool without slipping or tripping over objects.

Required objects
Cooker (hob) or microwave, toaster, plate, knife for spreading butter, spoon for stirring beans, tin opener, pan or bowl for heating beans. Ingredients: tin of beans, cheese and bread.

Objects need to be accessible in the kitchen, ideally placed close to each other for ease of use. A pan needs to be suitable for the cooker or a bowl needs to be safe to use in the microwave. The tin opener needs to be sharp enough for its purpose, with handles which can be gripped so it can be manipulated around the tin.

Required social context
Cooking could be done by yourself. Interaction is not generally required unless you are sharing the kitchen space. It is typically expected that someone cooking will do so

Table 4.4 (Continued)

safely and clean up afterwards, particularly if it is a shared kitchen. Noise levels can be a consideration if the cooking is happening very early or late in the day.

Required temporal context

Cooking lunch generally happens once a day in the middle of the day. Cooking in general can happen more frequently. It is often seen as a necessity to maintain health and a budget. It needs to happen before you can eat. Making a meal such as this would take under 30 mins.

Section 3: Steps and actions

Required sequence

Steps	Actions
Get utensils (plate, knife, spoon, cheese grater, pan, tin opener) These steps are somewhat flexible in order, each taking a few seconds.	Looking for utensils Choosing utensils Reaching for, grasping and lifting utensils Placing utensils on kitchen bench
Get ingredients (beans, bread, butter, cheese) These steps are somewhat flexible in order, each taking a few seconds.	Looking for ingredients Reaching for the fridge door handle Pulling the fridge door handle Opening the fridge Reaching for, grasping, choosing and lifting ingredients (one at a time) Placing ingredients on kitchen bench Closing the fridge door (same actions involved for getting beans from a cupboard)
Open beans This step is fixed if the beans are in a tin that requires a tin opener, as the opener needs to be used in a specific way to function. It is flexible if the beans are in a ring-pull can or a plastic container. This step takes less than 30 seconds.	Reaching, grasping, lifting tin opener Placing tin opener on the rim of the tin of beans Squeezing the tin opener together to close on the rim Twisting the handle of the opener to cut open the tin Opening the tin opener to release the tin Placing the open tin on the bench Gripping the tin lid and folding it back
Pour beans into pan Pouring beans is a fixed step, although a utensil could be used to scoop out the beans. This takes a few seconds. Using a pan and cooker is flexible as the beans could be heated in a microwave.	Reaching, grasping and lifting the open tin Tipping the beans into the pan Shaking the tin to remove all beans

Table 4.4 (Continued)

Steps	Actions
Heat beans Some parts of this step are fixed, such as turning on the cooker before beans can be heated and turning it off at the end. Stirring frequency is flexible. This takes a few minutes. A microwave could be used as an alternative.	Reaching, grasping and lifting the pan onto the cooker Grasping and twisting the cooker knob to turn it on Stirring the beans to heat through Noticing when beans are bubbling and hot enough Turning off the cooker when heated Placing the pan off the cooker on a heat-proof surface
Cook toast Some parts of this step are fixed, such as putting the bread in the toaster before turning it on. This takes around a minute. It can be flexible if a grill is used. Cooking toast can happen before heating the beans.	Finding the bread on the bench Opening the bread packet Reaching, grasping and lifting a slice of bread Placing the bread in the toaster (and letting it go) Pushing the toaster button to start toasting Reaching, grasping and lifting the toast when cooked Placing toast on the plate Finding butter and opening it Choosing a knife and using it to get some butter Spreading the butter on the toast and holding the toast steady
Grate cheese Some parts of this step are fixed, such as opening the cheese packet before grating the cheese. This takes around a minute. It can be flexible if pre-grated cheese is used or if a food processor is used to grate the cheese. This could happen before cooking toast or heating beans.	Finding the cheese grater and cheese Opening the cheese packet using scissors or pulling the ends of the packet apart Holding the cheese and the cheese grater (one in each hand) Using hands together to push the cheese onto the grater, moving the cheese up and down to grate it Stopping grating when enough cheese is grated
Assemble beans on toast with cheese Typically, the toast would be on the bottom of the plate with beans on top and cheese on top of that, although beans and cheese may be swapped. The toast could also be separate from the beans and cheese and dipped into the bowl. Cleaning and putting away may happen after eating. Assembling the meal takes under a minute.	Reaching, grasping and lifting the pan of heated beans Moving the pan to the plate of toast Tilting the pan so the beans fall on the toast Using a spoon to scrape out all the beans Placing the pan down on a heat-proof surface Reaching, grasping and choosing the grated cheese Sprinkling the grated cheese on top of the beans Lifting the plate and transporting it to the table to eat Cleaning and putting away the remaining ingredients and utensils

Table 4.4 (Continued)

Section 4: Body functions and structures

Making beans on toast with cheese.*

*Please note that all body functions were considered. These lists were thought to have a significant potential impact on doing this activity, although you may think of others.

Mental functions

Orientation	Knowing about making lunch in a kitchen at an appropriate time
Energy and drive	Having the motivation and interest in making lunch
Memory	Remembering the steps in the activity and the order in which to do things
Perception	Finding objects in the kitchen; recognising when something is hot
Higher cognitive functions	Judging when beans are hot; knowing that cooker needs to be turned on and off

Sensory Functions and Pain

Seeing	Locating the utensils and ingredients
Touch	Feeling when something is hot (pan/cooker) or sharp (knife/tin)

Cardiovascular, haematological, immunological and respiratory functions

Heart	Having the endurance to stand in the kitchen for the time needed to cook the meal

Neuromuscular and movement-related functions

Mobility of joints	Being able to hold utensils and ingredients
Muscle power	Having the muscle power to a lift pan of beans and to squeeze the tin opener to open the tin
Movement functions	Holding the tin and manipulating the tin opener, holding the bread while buttering it, walking with the plate to the table

For someone new to activity analysis, it is important to complete the template on many different activities and in as much detail as possible to develop knowledge and understanding. As you gain experience, this analysis often becomes integrated into everyday thinking and reasoning, and filling in a form to capture these considerations becomes less important. Be careful not to jump into the analysis without the template to structure your considerations too quickly, as this is likely to mean key aspects could be missed.

OCCUPATIONAL PERFORMANCE ANALYSIS

Occupational performance analysis is a way of *observing* a person perform an occupation to determine what is supporting or hindering them being able to participate to his/her desired level. An occupational performance analysis is *structured*, *detailed* and always placed *in the context* of the occupations a person wants or needs to perform (Chard and Mesa, 2017).

You observe and do occupational performance analyses to help you understand the people (what they do, why they do it, how they do it), the places where they do their occupations (e.g. home, workplace, school or community) and how aspects such as a person's health, physical, social, societal, economic or political restrictions can impact on his/her roles and way of life (Chard and Mesa, 2017). An occupational performance analysis will assist you to gather sufficient and relevant details to support your reasoning for interventions.

When planning your observation and occupational performance analysis, you need to be specific about what it is that you need to find out. Observing things which are not a priority for the person could be a waste of time (yours and the person's). Chapter 8 explores what you can do to collaboratively develop an occupational profile of a person and determine what is important for them (and relevant others). This means you can be specific about the occupation(s) you need to observe. For example, you may receive a referral where the concern raised is about 'personal hygiene'. You will need to find out more about this to plan your observation as you cannot observe 'personal hygiene'. You can, however, observe a person combing his/her hair or brushing his/her teeth, which might be the important elements for a person's personal hygiene (Chard and Mesa, 2017).

Analysis of observations can take many different forms. Table 4.5 (also downloadable from www.routledge.com/9781138238480) illustrates one example of an occupational performance analysis template which was developed by Dancza and Head (2013) and is non-standardised, although it is based on the work of Anne Fisher and shares a common language with standardised measures she has developed (e.g. Assessment of Motor and

Table 4.5 Occupational performance analysis template

Priority occupation you are observing:
Date and time of observation: **Persons present:**

Satisfaction with Overall Occupational Performance
Person's perspective (captured via interview) – How important is *this* occupation for the person? – What is the purpose of this occupation? – How satisfied is the person at present with his/her performance in *this* occupation?
Notes:

Table 4.5 (Continued)

Social support's perspective (if applicable; captured via interview)
– How important is *this* occupation for relevant people in a close relationship to the person (e.g. family member, partner, friend, carer, support worker)?   – What is the purpose of this occupation?   – How satisfied is the supporter(s) at present with the person's performance in *this* occupation?
Notes:
Key stakeholder(s) perspective (if applicable; captured via interview)   – How important is *this* occupation for the any relevant stakeholders (e.g. other professionals involved with this person, service setting requirements)?   – What is the purpose of this occupation?   – How satisfied is the relevant stakeholder(s) at present with the person's performance in *this* occupation?
Notes:

Overall Quality of Performance (please circle)		
Physical effort or clumsiness	Efficiency (disorganisation) in use of time, space or objects	Social appropriateness
No increase	Efficient	Appropriate
Minimal	Minimal	Minimal disruption
Moderate	Moderate	Moderate disruption
Marked	Marked	Marked disruption
Safety (risk of personal injury/ environmental damage)	Need for assistance (independence)	
Safe – Minimal – Moderate – Marked	Independent – Occasional – Frequent-Constant	

Social Interaction Skills	
Skill item Please indicate in the adjacent box (*) if a skill item caused significant challenge to the occupational performance.	Description of key observations
Initiating and terminating social interaction – Approaches/starts – Concludes/disengages	
Produces social interaction – Produces speech – Gesticulates – Speaks fluently	

Table 4.5 (Continued)

Physically supporting social interaction – Turns toward – Looks – Places self – Touches – Regulates		
Shaping content of social interaction – Questions – Replies – Discloses – Expresses emotions – Disagrees – Thanks		
Maintaining flow of social interaction – Transitions – Time response – Times duration – Takes turns		
Verbally supporting social interaction – Matches language – Clarifies – Acknowledges/encourages – Empathises		
Adapting social interaction – Heeds – Accommodates – Benefits		

Motor Skills		
Skill item Please indicate in the adjacent box (*) if a skill item caused significant challenge to the occupational performance.		**Description of key observations**
Body position – Stabilises – Aligns – Positions		

Table 4.5 (Continued)

Obtaining and holding objects – Reaches – Bends – Grips – Manipulates – Coordinates		
Moving self and objects – Moves – Lifts – Walks – Transports – Calibrates – Flows		
Sustaining performance – Endures – Paces		

Process Skills	
Skill item Please indicate in the adjacent box (*) if a skill item caused significant challenge to the occupational performance.	Description of key observations
Sustaining performance – Paces (already noted under motor skills) – Attends – Heeds	
Applying knowledge – Chooses – Uses – Handles – Inquires	
Temporal organisation – Initiates – Continues – Sequences – Terminates	

(Continued)

Table 4.5 (Continued)

Organising space and objects – Searches/locates – Gathers – Organises – Restores – Navigates		
Adapting performance – Notices/responds – Adjusts – Accommodates – Benefits		

Environmental Context
Describe the social context where the occupation took place: – Ambiance e.g. rushed or calm, hostile, sympathetic – Degree of familiarity e.g. routine or novel tasks – Language e.g. complexity, pace – Interaction e.g. communication between people – Norms and rules e.g. explicit and implied
Notes:
Describe the physical space where the occupation was performed (consider using a plan and description): – Visual e.g. lighting, distractions – Auditory e.g. noise level – Tactile e.g. textures of materials – Movement e.g. space to move, flow of movement – Temperature
Notes:
List any equipment/tools/objects which were used: – Provide a physical description of key objects – What is the meaning of the object to the person (if relevant)
Notes:

Process Skills, Fisher and Bray Jones, 2012; School Assessment of Motor and Process Skills, Fisher, Bryze Jones, Hume and Griswold, 2007; Evaluation of Social Interaction, Fisher and Griswold, 2015). Table 4.6 provides an example of a completed occupational performance analysis for a young adult named Lee (who has a diagnosis of Down's syndrome) who was observed making his lunch of beans on toast with cheese. Lee is a pseudonym, as are all the names in this book. It is important, however, that when you complete your own occupational performance analysis, notes and reports, that you use the person's correct first and last names.

Table 4.6 Occupational performance analysis: Lee Bristol

Priority occupation you are observing: Making and eating lunch consisting of baked beans on toast with grated cheese and a glass of juice

Date and time of observation: Friday 10/1/17, (interview 11:00–12:30) and observation 12:30–1:00, Lee's one-bedroom flat

Persons present: Lee Bristol, Viktor Papir (social worker) and the occupational therapist

Satisfaction With Overall Occupational Performance
Lee's perspective (captured via interview)
Lee is motivated to develop his meal planning and preparation skills. He understands that eating well is important for his health and he wants to demonstrate that he is able to achieve this. He would also like to show his parents that he can cook for himself by preparing a meal for them.
The purpose of this occupation for Lee is so that he can remain independent in his flat and have more choice and control over his life. Although Lee likes to see his parents and he is happy to have a cleaner come in once a week, he does not want to rely on other people on a daily basis to manage his meals for him.
Lee reports that he is trying hard with cooking, but he finds he loses track of what he is doing. He tends to cook the same two things when he is on his own (beans on toast and beans on toast with cheese) and he said he would like more variety. He said he would like to cook pasta and sauce for his parents.
Lee's parent's perspectives (captured via telephone interview)
Lee's parents are keen for Lee to remain living independently. They want him to be able to plan and prepare his own meals as they are not able to continue the intensity of support they have been giving him.
The purpose of this occupation for Lee's parents is to know that Lee can take care of himself if they are not able to cook for him every night.
At present Lee's parents are happy that he can prepare his breakfasts, but do not feel he has the skills to prepare a hot snack or meal. They are concerned that he also does not appear to have a regular routine around eating.
Viktor's perspective (social worker, captured via interview)
Viktor feels it is necessary for Lee to develop his skills in planning and cooking his meals as his parents are finding it challenging to keep supporting him as frequently as they have been.

(Continued)

Table 4.6 (Continued)

The purpose of this occupation is that Viktor feels it is necessary for Lee to be able to safely cook for himself when needed so that he can remain living independently in his flat.

At present Viktor has concerns about Lee's cooking skills particularly relating to his safety and the variety of his meals. This has increased in importance as Lee's parents are not able to continue indefinitely with their current level of support for Lee due to their own health needs.

Overall Quality of Performance (please circle)		
Physical effort or clumsiness	Efficiency (disorganisation) in use of time, space or objects	Social appropriateness
No increase	Efficient	Appropriate
Minimal	Minimal	Minimal disruption
Moderate	Moderate	Moderate disruption
Marked	Marked	Marked disruption
Safety (risk of personal injury/ environmental damage) Safe – Minimal – Moderate – Marked	Need for assistance (independence) Independent – Occasional – Frequent – Constant	

Social Interaction Skills	
Skill item Please indicate in the adjacent box (*) if a skill item caused significant challenge to the occupational performance.	**Description of key observations**
Initiating and terminating social interaction – Approaches/starts – Concludes/disengages	OK to start and conclude the conversation – spoke to the occupational therapist and social worker during the task.
Produces social interaction – Produces speech – Gesticulates – Speaks fluently	Mumbled to himself – didn't interfere with his task performance.
Physically supporting social interaction – Turns toward – Looks – Places self – Touches – Regulates	Eye contact not always maintained. At times he looked down as he was speaking, but infrequently.

Table 4.6 (Continued)

Shaping content of social interaction		
– Questions		Asked appropriate questions when seeking help from the occupational therapist.
– Replies	*	Short delay in responding.
– Discloses		Thanked therapist appropriately when assistance provided.
– Expresses emotions		
– Disagrees		
– Thanks		
Maintaining flow of social interaction		
– Transitions		Some short pauses and hesitations before responding to questions.
– Times response	*	
– Times duration	*	At times answers were quite short.
– Takes turns	*	On two occasions Lee seemed to seek input regarding the suggestions he made but he did not wait for response.
Verbally supporting social interaction		
– Matches language		Lee spoke to the therapist using suitable words.
– Clarifies		A small amount of acknowledgement and encouragement from Lee but it did not interfere with the performance.
– Acknowledges/encourages		
– Empathises		
Adapting social interaction		
– Heeds		Able to maintain the social interaction so that he could complete the occupation.
– Accommodates	*	
– Benefits	*	Lee asked for assistance when needed. His mild problems with maintaining the flow of the social interaction did however persist, but not so that he was unable to complete the occupation.

Motor Skills	
Skill item Please indicate in the adjacent box (*) if a skill item caused significant challenge to the occupational performance.	Description of key observations
Body position	
– Stabilises	Occasional prop on the bench with his hand to steady himself when completing the task.
– Aligns	Persistently leant forward, resting body against the kitchen bench.
– Positions	Lee positioned himself too close to the kitchen bench. Interfered with his arm movements when making his lunch.

Table 4.6 (Continued)

Motor Skills		
Obtaining and holding objects − Reaches − Bends − Grips − Manipulates − Coordinates	 * * *	Many grip slips on the cheese grater as he held it to grate his cheese. Also slips on the tin as he used the can opener. Fumbled when using the can opener to open his tin of beans so that he was not able to remove the lid and the tin dropped to the ground. This fumbling occurred when he was using two hands.
Moving self and objects − Moves − Lifts − Walks − Transports − Calibrates − Flows	 *	Lee was able to lift the tin and pour the beans into the saucepan. Able to transport pan of beans to the cooker competently. Lee did not press the can opener together with enough force to open the tin. Lee demonstrated some jerky hand and wrist movements when grating the cheese, spreading his bread with butter and opening the tin of beans.
Sustaining performance − Endures − Paces		Overall Lee was slow during the task performance.

Process Skills		
Skill item Please indicate in the adjacent box (*) if a skill item caused significant challenge to the occupational performance.		Description of key observations
Sustaining performance − Paces (already noted under motor skills) − Attends − Heeds		Overall pace for the task was slow. Lee kept to the task set, made his lunch and sat down to eat it, but he did not get himself a drink as previously arranged.
Applying knowledge − Chooses − Uses − Handles − Inquires	 * *	Couldn't remove lid of bean tin with a can opener − he used a sharp knife to stab the tin. This required the therapist to intervene as Lee was at risk of cutting himself. Didn't support bread as he was spreading it with butter − it slid over the chopping board where he had placed it. He also didn't handle the knife with care when attempting to open the tin.

Table 4.6 (Continued)

		Asked for information from the therapist but after short delay.
Temporal organisation – Initiates – Continues – Sequences – Terminates	* * * *	Frequent pauses: to start making his lunch; get out the beans from the cupboard; get out butter from the fridge. Prompting needed. Frequent pauses during steps: buttering his bread and grating the cheese. Prompting needed. Many sequences were illogical: not turning on the hob when heating the beans in his pan; buttering the bread then putting it in the toaster; trying to grate the cheese with the wrapper still on it. Went on too long: continued to spread his bread with butter after all of the bread was covered; continued to grate the cheese – whole 200g block.
Organising space and objects – Searches/locates – Gathers – Organises – Restores – Navigates	* * * *	Random searching strategy for finding the pan in the cupboard and the cutlery in the drawer. He needed to go to multiple places before finding each item. Lee placed the items in multiple work spaces. The kitchen bench had many items placed on it, with some close to the edge which were then knocked to the floor. Lee did not put away any of the items he used.
Adapting performance – Notices/responds – Adjusts – Accommodates – Benefits	* * * *	Did not notice that the beans were rapidly boiling in the pan. Didn't take the beans off the heat until prompted. Did not turn off the hob when he was finished cooking until prompted. Lee did not anticipate or prevent his motor and process skill problems and he did not alter the way he was doing the activity. However, he did respond when given the prompts by the therapist and he did benefit from this direction.

(Continued)

Table 4.6 (Continued)

Environmental Context

Describe the social context where the occupation took place:

Ambiance: Lee appeared comfortable in his own flat and the atmosphere was calm and supportive of Lee.

Degree of familiarity: Lee was very familiar with Viktor and was comfortable in his presence. This was the first meeting with the occupational therapist but Lee soon appeared comfortable with her presence.

Language: The occupational therapist and social worker matched Lee's language and spoke in a clear and slow pace.

Interaction: At first Lee was talking only with Viktor, but after a few minutes he was happy to answer the occupational therapist's questions as well. He was also comfortable to ask questions of both Viktor and the occupational therapist.

Norms and rules: On entering the flat, Lee offered a cold drink to both Viktor and the occupational therapist as this was something which Viktor had been working on with Lee. He was making some of the rules of social interaction explicit as Lee did not always pick these up independently. However, with instruction, Lee could recall and use these strategies.

Describe the physical space where the occupation was performed (consider using a plan and description):

Small kitchen, electric cooker and oven, fridge and sink.

Cupboards above and below a small workbench. In the cupboards, Lee had a range of plates, bowls, mugs and many pots and pans. Cutlery and utensils were divided between three kitchen drawers which also contained other items such as plastic bags and paper.

Many objects on the workbench – a large stack of newspapers and magazines (close to the cooker), empty containers and cartons, and a pile of DVDs and CDs. Also, food items on the bench such as cereal packets, biscuits, crisps and soda bottles.

Visual: Lighting was from a florescent light in the kitchen which was adequate for the task. The workbench was a dark laminate.

Auditory: The noise level was low.

Tactile: The kitchen floor was tiled and could be slippery.

Movement: Comfortable space for one person in the u-shaped kitchen.

Temperature: The temperature was warm but not uncomfortable.

List any equipment/tools/objects which were used.

- The can opener was metal with thin handles.
- The cheese grater was one flat surface with a handle on the top.
- Lee used a small saucepan with a metal handle to heat up his beans.
- Lee used a small, plastic chopping board to place his bread on as he was spreading it with butter.
- Lee used a two-slice toaster to toast his bread.
- The knife Lee used to spread his toast was a regular butter knife. The knife Lee used to assist in opening the tin was a bread knife.

STEP-BY-STEP GUIDE TO COMPLETING AN OCCUPATIONAL PERFORMANCE ANALYSIS

SATISFACTION WITH OVERALL OCCUPATIONAL PERFORMANCE

The first section asks about the *perceptions of the person, relevant social support(s) and other stakeholder(s)* about this specific priority occupation. For example, in Table 4.6, Lee's views are captured along with his parents' views (social support) and his social worker's views (another stakeholder). Notes gathered here can support your interpretations of how the occupation was performed. This involves you asking each person about:

1   The importance of the occupation (How meaningful is the occupation to the person and others?)
2   The purpose of the occupation (Why is the occupation undertaken?)
3   How the occupation was performed (Was the occupation carried out in the usual way for the person? How satisfied was he/she with his/her performance?)

These responses can be summarised to form part of an occupational therapy report. Chapter 9 focuses on documentation and contains the completed occupational therapy report for Lee in Appendix 9.1.

OVERALL QUALITY OF PERFORMANCE

The second section of the occupational performance analysis is where you can record the *overall quality of performance*. This is a non-standardised assessment, based on the observations you make of the *entire occupational performance*. It can be used as a baseline so you can monitor if this performance changes over time. It can also be used to support your reasoning and selection of intervention approach (for example compensating for an occupational performance challenge if there is an imminent safety risk). To support consistency in rating the overall quality of performance, Table 4.7 provides a description of each rating. An example of how this can be reported is shown in Lee's report (see the appendix to Chapter 9).

Table 4.7 Rating scales for overall quality of performance

Physical effort or clumsiness	No increase	No evidence of a problem or impact on occupational performance resulting from increased effort or clumsiness
	Minimal	Possible or minor impact on occupational performance resulting from increased effort or clumsiness
	Moderate	Disruption, interference or interruption to the occupational performance from increased effort or clumsiness.
	Marked	Increased effort or clumsiness which results in unacceptable outcome

(Continued)

Table 4.7 (Continued)

Efficiency (disorganisation) in use of time, space or objects	Efficient	No evidence of a problem or impact on occupational performance resulting from disorganisation
	Minimal	Possible or minor impact on occupational performance resulting from disorganisation
	Moderate	Disruption, interference or interruption to the occupational performance resulting from disorganization
	Marked	Disorganisation which results in an unacceptable outcome
Social appropriateness	Appropriate	No evidence of a problem or impact on occupational performance resulting from social interactions
	Minimal disruption	Possible or minor impact on occupational performance resulting from social interactions
	Moderate disruption	Disruption, interference or interruption to the occupational performance resulting from social interactions
	Marked disruption	Social interactions which result in an unacceptable outcome
Safety (risk of personal injury/ environmental damage)	Safe	No safety concern during the occupational performance
	Minimal	A safety concern which had a potential or minor impact on occupational performance
	Moderate	A safety concern which disrupted, interfered with or interrupted the occupational performance
	Marked	A safety concern which requires the occupational perfomance to be stopped or results in an unacceptable outcome
Need for assistance (independence)	Independent	No evidence of a problem or impact on occupational performance which required assistance
	Occasional	Possible or minor impact on occupational performance which required infrequent asssitance
	Frequent	Disruption, interference or interruption to the occupational performance which required numerous or regular assistance
	Constant	Occupational performance which required continuous assistance

Adapted from Fisher (2009). Reprinted with permission.

RECORDING OBSERVATIONS OF ACTIONS (SKILL ITEMS)

The occupational performance analysis then directs you to consider the person's social interaction, motor and process skills (actions) as they do the occupation. Each skill item has an explanation which is detailed in the guidance notes contained in Appendix 4.1. These *skill items relate to the actions and steps* described in the activity analysis.

It is important to make detailed notes against each of the skill items about what you saw during the observation. This will support your analysis and recording of the person's strengths and challenges carrying out this occupation. There is a space beside each of the skill items to indicate which ones most impacted on the occupational performance. These skill items will form the clusters in the reporting of the observation (see Chapter 9 for a description of how to develop clusters and examples within Lee's completed report, provided in the appendix to that chapter).

ENVIRONMENTAL CONTEXT

The final section of the occupational performance analysis guides you to record key features within the *environmental context* that the occupation took place. Prompts are included to consider the social context, physical space, and qualities of the tools and objects used. Each of these factors potentially supported or hindered the occupational performance. Where appropriate, it may be useful to take photographs (with permission) of relevant aspects of the environment to make recommendations for interventions clear. It can also support the recording of outcomes if the physical environment was changed. Examples of how the environmental context was summarised in Lee's report is shown in the appendix to Chapter 9.

CHAPTER SUMMARY

Occupational therapy is concerned with the things people do to occupy their time. As occupations are fundamental to the work we do, it is important that we have the tools we need to effectively analyse, make sense of, and plan interventions in relation to occupations.

Occupational profiling is one way we can think about the range of occupations a person does and the priority areas on which we may focus. From this understanding of the important occupation(s) we can use activity analysis to help us consider the complexity and potential of someone doing this activity. This enriched understanding of the activity prepares us for doing an observation of the person *doing* the priority occupation. We consolidate our observations through completing an occupational performance analysis, which helps us determine where the strengths and challenges for the person lie. This is essential for us to use our reasoning and collaboratively plan interventions which will enhance a person's occupational performance.

These key tools of the occupational therapist will form the foundation for your skills in carrying out the occupational therapy process. As with any skill worth developing, it will take time and practice to get the most out of this learning. But as your experience grows, it does become quicker and a little easier, and it is definitely worth it!

APPENDIX 4.1

OCCUPATIONAL PERFORMANCE SKILLS INCLUDED IN THE OTIPM: SOCIAL INTERACTION, MOTOR AND PROCESS

Social interaction skills

Occupational performance skills that represent small, observable actions related to communicating and interacting with others in the context of daily life task performances that involve social interaction.

Initiating and terminating social interaction:

Approaches/starts – approaches or initiates interaction with the social partner in a manner that is socially appropriate

Concludes/disengages – effectively terminates the conversation or social interaction, brings to closure the topic under discussion, and disengages or says goodbye

Produces social interaction:

Produces speech – produces spoken, signed or augmentative (i.e., computer-generated) messages that are audible and clearly articulated

Gesticulates – uses socially appropriate gestures to communicate or support a message

Speaks fluently – speaks in a fluent and continuous manner, with an even pace (not too fast, not too slow), and without pauses or delays during the message being sent

Physically supporting social interaction:

Turns toward – actively positions or turns the body and the face toward the social partner or the person who is speaking

Looks – makes eye contact with the social partner

Places self – positions oneself at an appropriate distance from the social partner during the social interaction

Touches – responds to and uses touch or bodily contact with the social partner in a manner that is socially appropriate

Regulates – does not demonstrate irrelevant, repetitive or impulsive behaviours that are not part of social interaction

Shaping content of social interaction:

Questions – requests relevant facts and information and asks questions that support the intended purpose of the social interaction

Replies – keeps conversation going by replying appropriately to questions and comments

Discloses – reveals opinions, feelings and private information about oneself or others in a manner that is socially appropriate

Expresses emotions – displays affect and emotions in a way that is socially appropriate

Disagrees – expresses differences of opinion in a socially appropriate manner

Thanks – uses appropriate words and gestures to acknowledge receipt of services, gifts or compliments

Maintaining flow of social interaction:

Transitions – handles transitions in the conversation or changes the topic without disrupting the ongoing conversation

Times response – replies to social messages without delay or hesitation and without interrupting the social partner

Times duration – speaks for a reasonable length of time given the complexity of the message sent

Takes turns – takes his/her turn and gives the social partner the freedom to take his/her turn.

Verbally supporting social interaction:

Matches language – uses a tone of voice, dialect and level of language that is socially appropriate and matched to the social partner's abilities and level of understanding

Clarifies – responds to gestures or verbal messages signalling that the social partner does not comprehend or understand a message and ensures that the social partner is 'following' the conversation

Acknowledges/encourages – acknowledges receipt of messages, encourages the social partner to continue interaction and encourages all social partners to participate in social interaction

Empathises – expresses a supportive attitude towards the social partner by agreeing with, empathizing with or expressing understanding of the social partner's feelings and experiences

Adapting social interaction:

Heeds – uses goal-directed social interactions focused toward carrying out and completing the intended purpose of the social interaction

Accommodates – prevents ineffective or socially inappropriate social interaction

Benefits – prevents problems with ineffective or socially inappropriate social interaction from recurring or persisting

Adapted from Fisher (2009, pp. 153–171). Reprinted with permission.

Motor skills

Occupational performance skills that represent small, observable actions related to interacting with and moving task objects or oneself in the context of performing a daily life task. Commonly named in terms of type of task being performed (e.g., Activities of Daily Living [ADL] motor skills, school motor skills, work motor skills).

Body position:

Stabilises – moves through task environment and interacts with task objects without momentary propping or loss of balance

Aligns – interacts with task objects without evidence of persistent propping or persistent leaning

Positions – positions self an effective distance from task objects without evidence of awkward arm or body positions

Obtaining and holding objects:

Reaches – effectively extends the arm, and when appropriate, bends the trunk, to effectively grasp or place task objects that are out of reach

Bends – flexes or rotates the trunk as appropriate to the task when sitting down or when bending to grasp or place task objects that are out of reach

Grips – effectively pinches or grasps task objects such that the objects do not slip (e.g., from the person's fingers, from between the teeth)

Manipulates – uses dexterous finger movements, without evidence of fumbling, when manipulating task objects (e.g., manipulating buttons when buttoning)

Coordinates – uses two or more body parts together to manipulate and hold task objects without evidence of fumbling task objects or objects slipping from his/her grasp

Moving self and objects:

Moves – effectively pushes or pulls task objects along a supporting surface, pulls to open or pushes to close doors and drawers or pushes on wheels to propel a wheelchair

Lifts – effectively raises or lifts task objects without evidence of increased effort

Walks – during the task performance, ambulates on level surfaces without shuffling the feet, becoming unstable, propping or using assistive devices

Transports – carries task objects from one place to another while walking or moving in a wheelchair

Calibrates – uses movements of appropriate force, speed or extent when interacting with task objects (e.g., not crushing task objects, pushing a door with enough force that it closes)

Flows – uses smooth and fluid arm and wrist movements when interacting with task objects

Sustaining performance:

Endures – persists and completes the task without obvious evidence of physical fatigue, pausing to rest or stopping to catch his/her breath

Paces – maintains a consistent and effective rate or tempo of performance throughout the entire task

Note: Paces is both a motor skill and a process skill, but we evaluate it only once, based on the person's overall rate or tempo of task performance.

Process skills

Occupational performance skills that represent small, observable actions related to selecting, interacting with and using task objects; carrying out individual actions and steps; and modifying task performance to prevent problems of occupational performance from occurring or reoccurring in the context of performing a daily life task. Commonly named in terms of type of task being performed (e.g., ADL process skills, school process skills, work process skills).

Sustaining performance:

Paces – maintains a consistent and effective rate or tempo of performance throughout the entire task

Attends – does not look away from what he/she is doing, interrupting the ongoing task progression

Heeds – carries out and completes the task originally agreed upon or specified by another

Applying knowledge:

Chooses – selects necessary and appropriate type and number of tools and materials for the task, including the tools and materials that the person was directed to use (e.g., by a teacher) or specified he/she would use

Uses – applies tools and materials as they are intended (e.g., using a pencil sharpener to sharpen a pencil, but not to sharpen a crayon), and in a hygienic fashion

Handles – supports or stabilises task objects in an appropriate manner, protecting them from damage, slipping, moving or falling

Inquires – (a) seeks needed verbal or written information by asking questions or reading directions or labels, and (b) does not ask for information in situations where he/she was fully oriented to the task and environment and had immediate prior awareness of the answer

Temporal organisation:

Initiates – starts or begins the next action or step without hesitation

Continues – performs single actions or steps without interruptions such that once an action or task step is initiated, the individual continues without pauses or delays until the action or step is completed

Sequences – performs steps in an effective or logical order and with an absence of (a) randomness or lack of logic in the ordering, and/or (b) inappropriate repetition of steps

Terminates – brings to completion single actions or single steps without inappropriate persistence or premature cessation

Organising space and objects:

Searches/locates – looks for and locates tools and materials in a logical manner, both within and beyond the immediate environment

Gathers – collects related tools and materials into the same workspace, and regathers tools or materials that have spilled, fallen or been misplaced

Organises – logically positions or spatially arranges tools and materials in an orderly fashion within a single workspace, and between multiple appropriate workspaces, such that the workspace is not too spread out or too crowded

Restores – puts away tools and materials in appropriate places, and ensures that the immediate workspace is restored to its original condition

Navigates – moves the arm, body or wheelchair without bumping into obstacles when moving in the task environment or interacting with task objects

Adapting performance:

Notices/responds – responds appropriately to (a) nonverbal task-related cues (e.g., heat, movement), (b) the spatial arrangement and alignment of task objects to one another and (c) cupboard doors or drawers that have been left open during the task performance

Adjusts – effectively (a) goes to a new workspace(s); (b) moves tools and materials out of the current workspace; and (c) adjusts knobs, dials or water taps to overcome problems with ongoing task performance

Accommodates – prevents ineffective task performance

Benefits – prevents problems with task performance from recurring or persisting

Adapted from Fisher, A. G. (2009). *Occupational Therapy Intervention Process Model: A model for planning and implementing top–down, client-centered, and occupation-based interventions* (pp. 153–171). Ft. Collins, CO: Three Star Press. Reprinted with permission.

REFERENCES

American Occupational Therapy Association (2014) 'Occupational therapy practice framework: Domain and process (3rd edition)'. *American Journal of Occupational Therapy*, 68, S1–S48.

Chard G, Mesa S (2017) 'Analysis of occupational performance: Motor, process and social interaction skills'. In: M Curtin, J Adams, M Egan, eds, *Occupational therapy for people experiencing illness, injury or impairment: Promoting occupation and participation.* 7th edn. Edinburgh: Elsevier, pp. 217–243.

Christiansen C, Townsend E (2014) *Introduction to occupation: The art of science and living.* 2nd edn. Essex, UK: Pearson.

Creek J (2010) *The core concepts of occupational therapy: A dynamic framework for practice.* London, UK: Jessica Kingsley Publishers.

Dancza K, Head J (2013) 'Occupational performance analysis template'. *MPLHS2ENC enabling occupational change*. Canterbury Christ Church University. Unpublished.

Fisher AG (2009) *Occupational therapy intervention process model: A model for planning and implementing top-down, client centred, and occupation-based interventions*. Fort Collins, CO: Three Star Press.

Fisher AG, Bray Jones K (2012) *Assessment of motor and process skills. Volume 1: Development, standardization, and administration manual*. 8th edn. Fort Collins, CO: Three Star Press.

Fisher AG, Bryze Jones K, Hume V, Griswold L (2007) *School AMPS: School version of the assessment of motor and process skills*. 2nd edn. Fort Collins, CO: Three Star Press, Inc.

Fisher AG, Griswold L (2015) *Evaluation of social interaction*. 2nd edn. Fort Collins, CO: Three Star Press.

Head J, Gray F, Dancza K (2014) 'Activity analysis worksheet'. *MPLHS2CAF concepts and frameworks of occupational therapy*. Canterbury Christ Church University. Unpublished.

Mackenzie L, O'Toole G (2011) *Occupation analysis in practice*. West Sussex, UK: Wiley-Blackwell.

Pierce DE (2003) *Occupation by design: Building therapeutic power*. Pennsylvania: F.A. Davis.

World Federation of Occupational Therapists (2012–last update) *What is occupational therapy?* [Homepage of World Federation of Occupational Therapists], [Online]. Available: www.wfot.org/AboutUs/AboutOccupationalTherapy/ WhatisOccupationalTherapy.aspx [October 22, 2016].

World Health Organisation (WHO) (2001) *The international classification of functioning, disability and health (ICF)*. Geneva: WHO. Available: www.who.int/classifications/icf/ en/ [October 22, 2016].

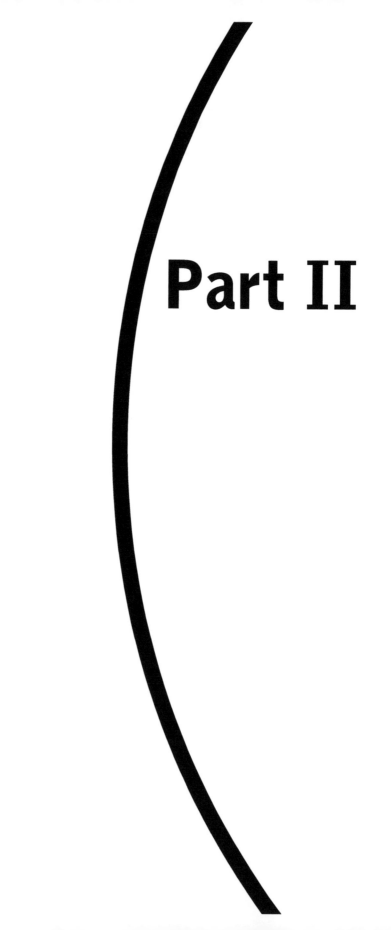

Part II

STEP-BY-STEP GUIDE TO THE OCCUPATIONAL THERAPY PROCESS

OVERVIEW

Part II (Chapters 5–13) guides student's practice learning through the step-by-step implementation of the occupational therapy process. We apply the theories and tools from Part I of this book and follow the Occupational Therapy Intervention Process Model (OTIPM; Fisher, 2009) as the framework. Each chapter focuses on part of the model with practical examples of how to enact this process in practice learning situations. The OTIPM (Fisher, 2009) was selected as it focuses on occupation at each step of the process. This model can be used with other occupational therapy models (see Chapter 11), which is important as students and practice areas often use a range of resources. In each chapter, guidance is offered for both students and educators.

Through using the OTIPM (Fisher, 2009) from beginning to end, it offers students and educators a coherent journey though the occupational therapy process. As mentioned in Chapter 1, at times this might seem prescriptive, particularly when we explore the use of occupational performance analysis as a key assessment tool and a way to structure our professional reasoning and reporting. Our experience developing the Professional Learning through Useful Support (PLUS) Framework (described in Chapter 14) has shown that when students are learning about these important concepts, they need a firm foundation which they can logically follow. Without this foundation, it is more difficult for students to appropriately select which models and tools to use. However, once they feel confident in an occupational therapy process, they can adapt, change and deviate from this theory foundation and set of tools as their learning develops and the situation requires.

Our advice is to use these chapters flexibly to suit your own practice learning context. Any decisions about which theory or tool to use, however, should be carefully made so that the coherence of the occupational therapy process and theoretical perspectives are maintained.

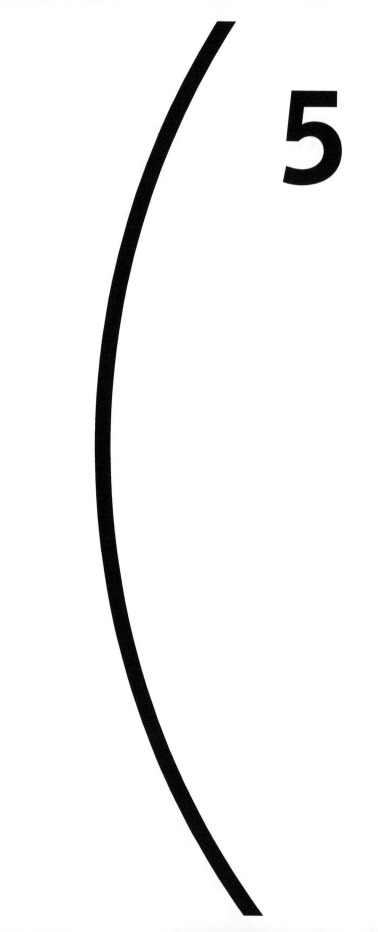

5

CHAPTER 5
PREPARING FOR PLACEMENT
Jodie Copley and Karina Dancza

INTENDED CHAPTER OUTCOMES

By the end of this chapter, readers will have an overview of:

- Preparation that is useful for students, including what can be done before placement begins, settling into the placement, planning learning and explaining the role of the occupational therapist in the setting
- Preparation that is useful for educators, including developing student orientation resources for a smooth beginning, creating a placement timeline and schedule and considering personal skill development needs for supervision

INTRODUCTION

Preparation affects the practice learning experience of both students and educators. Despite its importance, preparation can often be rushed as people are busy and it becomes a priority only in the preceding few weeks before the placement starts. This chapter aims to help students and educators make the most of this valuable time. It is divided into two sections: the first section is designed for students and recommends a structure for their preparation and suggestions for making the most of placement learning. The second section offers advice for educators in preparing for student placement.

Part of the preparation for educators involves identifying the ways in which they can help students settle into the placement and carry out the occupational therapy process. In this chapter, and for the remainder of this book, we will offer ideas for materials and opportunities that educators can prepare for students ahead of time which relate specifically to their context (such as report examples). Places where we think setting specific examples are useful are indicated by the phrase "educator examples here". These were summarised in Appendix 1.1 at the beginning of this book.

ADVICE FOR STUDENTS: PREPARATION FOR PLACEMENT

Receiving news that you have your placement allocation can be an exciting, if somewhat daunting, time for you. One of your main challenges is trying to prepare for the unknown. A good place to start is from the certainties you do know. For example, you know:

- That you will be expected to consider the occupational therapy role and its relationship to models of occupational therapy practice and the occupational therapy process
- What you have learned thus far and where you would like to further develop your skills and knowledge
- That you may need to work with a student peer
- That you will need to introduce yourself and explain your role
- That you will need to understand the range of occupations of the people you are working with

Each of these areas will be explored in this section.

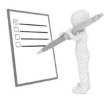

ACTIVITY

Try to arrange a pre-placement phone call and/or visit to the placement site. Check with your university placement coordinator first, but you may wish to ask about:

- **Practical information** such as placement location, transport, parking, start and finish time, uniform, lunch facilities and first-day arrangements
- **Information about the population you will be working with** such as age range, specific disabilities/conditions/life situations and types of occupations commonly encountered
- **Information about the service** such as the purpose, funding arrangements, team members, clinical pathways and average time spent with clients
- **Pre-reading or revision** you could do before the placement, for example, reviewing interview techniques you have learnt at university or reading literature on interventions relevant to this client group

RECOMMENDED PRELIMINARY READING

These texts provide you with general information about occupational therapy and some of the common models used in practice. As a starting point, we suggest that you revisit occupational therapy theory from Chapter 3. For more detail on the Occupational Therapy Intervention Process Model, see Fisher (2009) and for the other occupational therapy models, see Turpin and Iwama (2011).

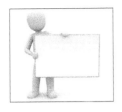

EDUCATOR EXAMPLES HERE:
RECOMMENDED PRELIMINARY READING

– Ask your educator to suggest any key recommended texts relevant for this placement setting.

PLANNING YOUR LEARNING

Reflect on your current skills before you start placement so that you can use and enhance your strengths, and focus on your learning needs. To assist with this, complete the checklist in Table 5.1. During your placement, ensure you understand how you will be evaluated through reading the placement paperwork and seeking support from your educators or placement coordinator. You are also encouraged to revisit Table 5.1 during your placement so you can use it to inform your placement reflections, learning objectives and evaluation.

Table 5.1 Self-reflection checklist for students

Learning and reflection

Desired attributes	Reflection questions for students
Self-directed learner and knowledge seeker	Do I naturally seek knowledge or wait to be told? Do I use existing resources? Do I ask questions and clarify when I am unsure?
Displays insight into strengths and weaknesses	What do I consider to be my strengths and challenges coming into this placement? What are my learning goals? How might I meet these?
Seeks out feedback	How do I find out how I am progressing? What questions might I ask to obtain feedback? When is the best time to do this?
Recognises own and educator's needs	How do I reflect on situations by myself? With my educator? How do I keep track of the needs of my educator? For example, is she/he pressured for time? Does she/he need me to take more responsibility for routine tasks? Do I need to take initiative to keep her/him informed?
Applies theory to practice	What theories do I need to know? How is theory applied to practice in this setting? How do I demonstrate my clinical reasoning?

Self-management

Desired attributes	Reflection questions for students
Demonstrates initiative	What do I notice about routines and procedures here? How can I demonstrate initiative here? What am I encouraged/not encouraged to do independently in this setting?

(Continued)

Table 5.1 (Continued)

Well organised and manages time	Am I naturally organised? Do I pick up on details? Am I systematic in my approach to tasks? Do I start tasks promptly or procrastinate? Do I manage my time well across the day/week? How can I improve this?

Professional behaviour and interaction

Desired attributes	*Reflection questions for students*
Presents professionally	How might I demonstrate professionalism in this environment? What does professional communication look like here?
Adapts to the agency environment	What do I need to do to "fit in" within this environment? What is important in terms of the social dynamics and team functioning in this workplace? What do others expect of the occupational therapy role?
Interacts well with staff and clients	What opportunities do I have for interaction? What do I need to consider when interacting with staff? How do I handle feedback from others?
Enthusiastic	In terms of my personality, how do I demonstrate my interest and enthusiasm for what I am doing?

Adapted from Thomas and Rodger (2011, p. 44).

WORKING IN COLLABORATION WITH ANOTHER OCCUPATIONAL THERAPY STUDENT

During your placement, you may have the opportunity to work with a student peer. You will have some projects which you undertake together and others in which you will take the lead and work independently. Both types of working will need to be negotiated and you will benefit from both. To make the most of working together, it is important to share your strengths and the areas in which you would like support.

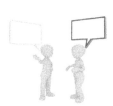

ACTIVITY

Consider the following questions and use them as a basis for discussion with your peer in your first few days of placement:

– What strengths will you bring to the placement?
– In which areas would you like support to improve your skills?
– How might you be able to support the learning of your student colleague?

INTRODUCING YOURSELF IN THE PLACEMENT

In your first few days on placement you will need to introduce yourself and talk to the staff members and clients about your role as an occupational therapy student. If you are on a role-emerging placement, this will be an ongoing process as people will understand your role through *observing what you do*. As there is likely to be no established role for an occupational therapist, you will need to build relationships with the community and clients and try to understand their occupational needs.

In both role-established and role-emerging placements, when talking about the role of occupational therapy, try to give an overview as well as some specific examples related to your setting. For example, you might say:

> "Occupational therapists are concerned with how you 'occupy' your time. What you do (or your occupations) affects your health and well-being. For example, in a work context, we are concerned with *how* you complete the tasks you need to, want to or are expected to do in your role as a worker. We might look at:
>
> – *How* you can get to work on time and work the required hours
> – *How* you organise your daily tasks for time effectiveness and endurance across the day
> – *How* you manage each of the work tasks required
> – *How* you participate in team activities in the workplace"

Be aware that the staff members and clients within the setting are experts in *what* they do. You will need to work in partnership as they know what is important (the occupations) and the environment far better than you do.

When explaining your role to clients, you will need to consider the language and level of detail you provide. For example, when working with children in a school setting, be prepared with a short statement to describe your role and again consider examples that are relevant for the classroom or setting you are in. For example, you might say:

> "I am here to help you do the tasks that you need to do at school, like organising your things so you don't lose them, or helping you do your school work or playing games and sports. We can work together as 'problem solvers' (or detectives) to find ways to do the things you want to or need to do."

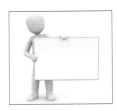

EDUCATOR EXAMPLES HERE: INTRODUCING YOURSELF

– Ask your educator for any key points that you need to be aware of when explaining your role in the placement context.

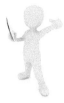

ACTIVITY
....

Create your own phrases to explain your role to:

– Clients and family members
– Other professionals
– Managers
– Other staff members

You may find that other staff members would like you to present to the whole team about the role of occupational therapy. An example of a presentation to teachers is available to download from www.routledge.com/9781138238480. The overall explanation of occupational therapy would be the same in any setting (as fundamentally occupational therapy is about occupation and its relationship to health and well-being), but your examples will need to be adapted to your placement context.

OCCUPATIONS OF THOSE YOU ARE WORKING WITH

When thinking about and explaining your role, it is important to keep focused on the clients' *occupations*. Examples of school occupations are listed in Table 5.2. For your placement preparation it will be useful to create your own table and populate it with example occupations that are relevant to the people you will be working with. Remember to think about a range of occupations such as self-care, leisure and productive occupations.

Table 5.2 Sample occupations for school

Occupations	Example tasks
Doing schoolwork	Maths – using rulers, compasses and maths blocks
	Science – using equipment and recording experiments
	English – writing stories, using the computer and completing worksheets
	Art – drawing and painting; using scissors, glue and craft supplies
	Sport – running, jumping, climbing, dancing, ball games
Being in the classroom	Listening to and following directions, answering questions, starting and finishing work, working with peers and adults, participating in group discussions and "carpet time"

Table 5.2 (Continued)

Occupations	Example tasks
Doing school routines	Waiting in line, roll call, cleaning the board, taking messages to different classrooms/ the office, participating in assembly
Looking after oneself	Washing hands, using the toilet, blowing nose, putting on shoes and socks, changing for sport, eating lunch and snacks, opening packets, pouring liquids and drinking, hanging up a jacket, and putting bag away
Organising oneself	Getting together materials, placing items so they are accessible on the desk, tidying up, putting rubbish in the bin, and packing and unpacking a school bag
Moving around the school	Getting to classes, walking/moving around the classroom and in the playground, carrying items between classes and moving chairs
Socialising and leisure	Playing on equipment in the playground, throwing/ kicking balls, skipping rope, pretend play, reading, playing on the computer, card games, and talking with peers and adults

ADVICE FOR EDUCATORS: PREPARATION FOR PLACEMENT

Preparing for a student placement involves the creation of a map to guide the student's progress throughout the placement. Ideally, this process is organised and structured enough to allow a gradual scaffolding of student responsibility and autonomy as the student gains skills and confidence, but flexible enough to respond to unpredictable events.

PLANNING THE PLACEMENT

Preparation begins long before the start of placement. As a potential educator, you will begin by engaging with the prospective student's university placement management team. Although the type and extent of resources available from the university will vary, you need to *clarify up-front the university's offerings*. Questions might include:

- What placement training workshops or resources are available?
- Is a university placement coordinator able to work with me directly to develop the placement in my setting?
- Can they point me towards established repositories of placement resources? For example, in Queensland, Australia, the Occupational Therapy Practice Education Collaborative of Queensland (OTPEC-Q) hosts an open-access website for this purpose at otpecq.group.uq.edu.au.

- Are there opportunities for role-established, role-emerging or project placements? (See the Glossary for a description of each placement type and Chapter 14 for a discussion of the value of each placement type.) What is the potential for elements of each?
- What are the university's requirements for student evaluation? What tool is used and when during the placement?

Consider which supervision model will provide the best fit for you, your organisation and the university program. For example:

- Is a one-to-one apprenticeship style supervision the best option?
- Would a collaborative placement with a small group of students (Bartholomai and Fitzgerald, 2007) better enable peer learning?
- Could a shared or inter-agency placement with another organisation (Fisher and Savin-Baden, 2002) offer interesting learning and networking opportunities?
- Would a multiple mentoring placement with several students and a group of educators (Copley and Nelson, 2012) provide opportunities for students to experience a range of supervision styles and part-time staff to experience being educators?
- If role-emerging or project placements are an option, who will be the long-arm and on-site supervisors or sponsors?
- Would a pair or group of students work better than an individual student so they can support each other?

Organisational change appears to be a constant in many service settings. Some educators are concerned that they will not be able to offer a suitable placement given the stress associated with such change. These opportunities do, however, help students learn about the realities of practice and develop skills in managing these challenges. Different placement models can help you and students manage in a fluctuating placement environment. For example, you may like to support students in a role-emerging setting such as a care home in your area or a school you support.

ACTIVITY

....

1   If you are in a role-established setting, is there a project or area of your practice you would like to develop? Could students help facilitate this?
2   Is there benefit to having two or more students in terms of peer learning and support? If so, how would the students' workload and responsibilities be organised?
3   Could you involve managers (who may not have a clinical caseload) or part time practitioners in student supervision? Make a list of activities the student could engage in to learn from them.

PREPARING THE PLACEMENT SITE TO RECEIVE THE STUDENT

Beyond the organisational requirements for having a student on-site, such as occupational health and safety procedures, you as an educator can also reflect on the *organisational culture* into which the student is entering. It is this organisational culture that determines, at a broad level, the expectations of the student in terms of communication, actions and behaviours.

As you are embedded in the organisational culture, you may not be consciously aware of the norms and expectations. Think back to when you first started within your role and what you needed to find out about the "unwritten rules". For example:

- Is it common for your colleagues to offer to make a hot drink for everyone when they go to the kitchen?
- Do you have specific mugs (and are people are offended if you use theirs)?
- Do people stop for lunch or eat at their desks?

Similarly, it is important to be aware of the communication expectations. For example:

- Do you need to keep certain staff members informed of your activities?
- Is this done through conversation or more formally through emails or meetings?
- How frequently is this required?
- Will the student(s) be expected to do the same?

It is important that you bring these aspects of the organisational culture into your conscious awareness, so that you can explain them to the students.

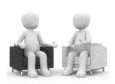

ACTIVITY
....

1   To help make explicit the "unwritten rules" of your setting, have a chat with a colleague from another setting to identify differences in communication and practices.
2   If planning a role-emerging or project placement, you as the long-arm supervisor should spend some time within the organisation talking to key staff members to work out what the student might need to know to "fit in".

ORIENTATION MATERIALS

If possible, a pre-placement visit from the student goes a long way to supporting her/his transition into the setting. Once the student begins the placement, her/his orientation may continue in some form throughout the first day or week, depending on the length of the placement.

Whilst verbal discussions are valuable, key orientation information should also be documented in an orientation package. Writing down the expectations allows you and the students to review the information at critical points and establish an agreed approach to the placement. Key aspects of this documentation are discussed in this section.

TIMETABLE

Make a clear timetable *for* the students in the first week and *with* the students thereafter. This may be in the form of a wall planner or electronic diary so that others can see the students' commitments. Providing an overall plan of the placement will allow students to see where their learning is headed and how they will take on increasing responsibility throughout the placement. Timetabling supervision sessions for the duration of the placement can be helpful for your scheduling and offers reassurance for students.

Figure 5.1 provides an example timetable for a *role-emerging placement, where students often spend more time planning and assessing* as there are few established structures for providing services in this context. This may look different in established placement settings where students can model their behaviour on occupational therapists. In these placements, students often undertake assessment and intervention earlier (e.g. an initial assessment process is established and an assessment form is available for the students to use or it is expected that the students support the running of an existing group).

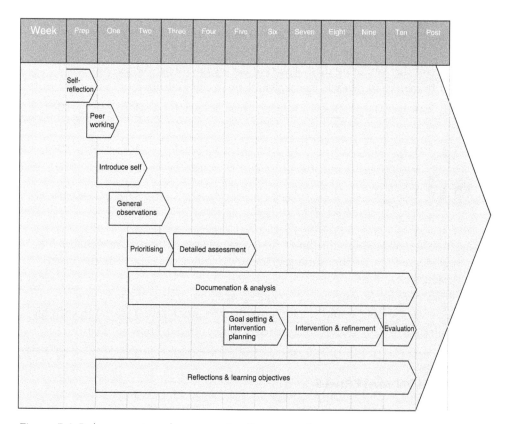

Figure 5.1 Role-emerging placement timeline example

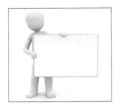

EDUCATOR EXAMPLES HERE: PLACEMENT
TIMELINE

– Create a placement timeline for the students that reflects the structure and length
  of the placement.

ORGANISATIONAL STRUCTURE AND PURPOSE

Describe the organisation for the student, including: how services are provided, management configurations, lines of reporting, how the service is funded, and its primary deliverables and intended outcomes. It is important that students understand the bigger picture of the organisation and see themselves as contributing to the service provision.

REQUIRED PROCEDURES AND PROCESSES

Make clear the daily or weekly procedures and processes the student will need to adhere to. These could include:

– Documentation requirements (see Chapter 9)
– Safety procedures
– Established communication systems and preferences such as in/out display boards
– Email and telephone protocols
– Formal face-to-face processes for communication such as ward rounds, case
  meetings or staff meetings.

STYLE AND LEVEL OF COMMUNICATION

The style and level of formality used when communicating with different staff members can be modelled within role-established placements (but still need to be emphasised explicitly to students). Introduce students to key people (clients, other professionals, family members, administration staff), modelling the style of communication that is appropriate in each case.

If you are the long-arm supervisor in a role-emerging or project placement, you may rely on close liaison with the on-site staff members to learn the usual communication methods and styles, so that you can support the students.

COMMUNICATION AND SUPERVISION WITH THE EDUCATOR

Expectations for the students' communication with you as the educator and engagement in supervision should be clearly documented. Consider including:

– Roles and responsibilities of different supervisors (e.g. long-arm and on-site
  supervisors, sponsor, primary supervisor and other members of the team)
– Frequency of supervision

- Preparation required by the student (e.g. generating an agenda, being prepared to present her/his reasoning for a client intervention, completing documentation drafts)
- Informal supervision opportunities before and after client encounters and the way these will be structured
- Expectations for student reflection (verbal and/or written, frequency and structure)
- Expectations for how the students should seek assistance and clarification (for example, saving up questions for weekly supervision, discussing with their student peer first, emailing urgent questions)

For many students, it is worth overtly inviting open and honest communication with you from early in the placement, as students may be concerned that expressing doubt or uncertainty will be viewed negatively. Open discussion gives you an opportunity to help them learn to express their questions and concerns in a constructive way.

FACILITATING TRANSITION INTO THE WORKPLACE

In addition to letting key staff members in your setting know that students are coming, it is important to prepare them for the role students may play and what to expect from them. The next section suggests some initiatives which can facilitate students' inclusion in your setting.

WORKSTATION

There may be limited choice in terms of space and logistical resources available for students, but where possible, think about their proximity to key staff members and how this might create informal interaction opportunities. Also consider the practicalities of access to a computer and electronic recording systems and somewhere to store personal belongings. This can help students feel welcomed and part of the team (Dancza, 2015).

OPPORTUNITIES TO PARTICIPATE

Consider opportunities for students' legitimate peripheral participation (Lave and Wenger, 1991), where they can be involved in a limited way in the events of the service. For example, in a hospital they might attend an outpatient clinic as an observer or helper; in a community service, there may be health promotion or open days students could assist with; and in a school environment there may be opportunities for them to join seasonal celebration activities.

Participating in these ways provides students with a "way in" to the shared organisational culture and the community of practice they are temporarily joining. It is particularly important for role-emerging placements, where students do not have an educator consistently on-site to ease their passage into the setting (Dancza, 2015).

PRESENT AS AN EDUCATOR–STUDENT TEAM

Present to others as an educator–student team in the early part of the placement. Going to meetings together with students can model to others that they have a valued contribution to make to the team. During the meeting, ask for the students' opinion or discuss options with them as this encourages the team to start viewing the students as connected with, and guided by, the occupational therapist.

These interaction opportunities subtly model to other staff members what they might be able to expect from students during future encounters. They can also instil confidence in the students as you have publicly communicated confidence in their abilities to the extent that is reasonable for the stage of their learning. Once other team members initiate communication with students, this further enhances their self-perception as being part of the team.

In role-emerging or project placements, opportunities to present as a student–educator team may be more difficult due to the limited amount of time the long-arm supervisor is on-site. Joint supervision opportunities with the on-site supervisor or sponsor can offer a way to present as an educator-student team.

CONSIDER YOUR OWN INFORMATION AND SKILL DEVELOPMENT NEEDS

It is important that, as an educator, you feel confident not only in your own practices as an occupation-centred therapist, but that you also feel equipped with teaching and learning techniques to effectively impart these practices to students. Chapter 14 contains some strategies to support your own learning which may be helpful to revisit during the placement preparation period. Learning is, however, an ongoing process and one of the benefits of hosting students is to learn together with them. Modelling your own ongoing professional development to students is a valuable lesson.

CHAPTER SUMMARY

Preparation is an important part of the success of any placement. It is worthwhile starting to prepare as early as possible so that orientation materials can be developed and schedules organised ahead of time. This chapter offers practical suggestions for students and educators to support placement preparation.

Students are encouraged to think about their learning needs, how they might work with a peer and how to introduce themselves in the setting. It is also important that students consider the occupations of the client group they will be working with.

Educators need contact with university placement co-ordinators to collaboratively design a suitable placement structure. This could be role-established, role-emerging or project placements with one or more students or supervisors. Orientation materials can include a timetable, information about the organisation, procedures and expectations for the student. Considering the space for students to work in, opportunities to participate in the setting and presenting as a student–educator team all facilitate the students' inclusion in the setting.

REFERENCES

Bartholomai S, Fitzgerald C (2007) 'The Collaborative Model of Fieldwork Education: Implementation of the model in a regional hospital rehabilitation setting'. *Australian Occupational Therapy Journal, 54,* S23–30.

Copley J, Nelson A (2012) 'Practice educator perspectives of multiple mentoring in diverse clinical settings'. *British Journal of Occupational Therapy, 75*(10), 456–462.

Dancza KM (2015) *Structure and uncertainty: The 'just right' balance for occupational therapy student learning on role-emerging placements in schools.* Doctor of Philosophy, The University of Queensland, Queensland, Australia.

Fisher A, Savin-Baden M (2002) 'Modernising fieldwork, part 2: Realising the new agenda'. *British Journal of Occupational Therapy, 65*(6), 275–282.

Fisher AG (2009) *Occupational Therapy intervention process model: A model for planning and implementing top-down, client centred, and occupation-based interventions.* Fort Collins, CO: Three Star Press.

Lave J, Wenger E (1991) *Situated learning: Legitimate peripheral participation.* Cambridge, UK: Cambridge University Press.

Thomas Y, Rodger S (2011) 'Successful role emerging placements: It is all in the preparation'. In: M Thew, M Edwards, S Baptiste, M Molineux, eds, *Role emerging occupational therapy: maximising occupation-focused practice.* West Sussex, UK.: Wiley-Blackwell, pp. 39–53.

Turpin M, Iwama MK (2011) *Using occupational therapy models in practice: A field guide.* London, UK: Churchill Livingstone Elsevier.

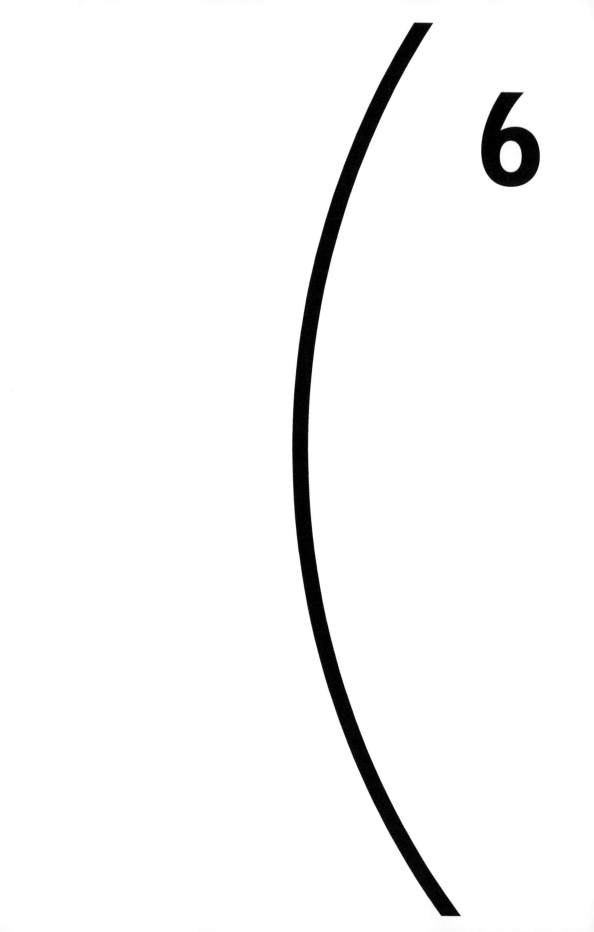

6

CHAPTER 6
ESTABLISHING THE CLIENT-CENTRED PERFORMANCE CONTEXT
Karina Dancza and Anita Volkert

INTENDED CHAPTER OUTCOMES

By the end of this chapter, readers will have an overview of:

- The first three aspects of the Occupational Therapy Intervention Process Model:
  1 Develop therapeutic rapport and work collaboratively with the client
  2 Establish the client-centred performance context
  3 Identify resources and limitations within the client-centred performance context
- Strategies for developing relationships with people in the placement context
- How to plan and do initial observations to gain an understanding of the placement context
- Reflective activities to capitalise on the learning that takes place in the first one to two weeks of placement

STAGES IN THE OTIPM

To structure your involvement and remain focused on the contribution of occupational therapy in the placement setting, it is important to work through an occupational therapy process. The remainder of Part II of this book will be following the process set out by the Occupational Therapy Intervention Process Model (OTIPM; Fisher, 2009). Each chapter will explore aspects of this process in detail, with examples of what you might do in your placement within each step. To remind you of where we are in the process, each chapter will start with the OTIPM diagram (Figure 6.1), highlighting the focus of the chapter. In this chapter, you are beginning the first part of the evaluation and goal-setting phase.

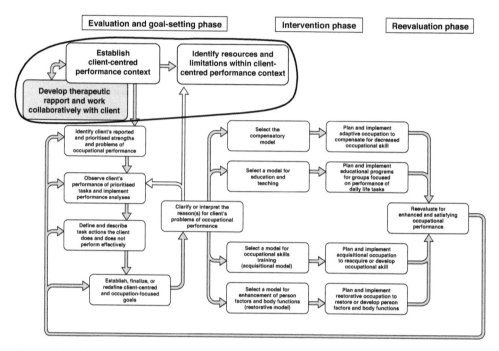

Figure 6.1 Schematic representation of the steps in the OTIPM: Establish client-centred performance context

Adapted from Fisher (2009). Available: www.innovativeotsolutions.com/content/wp-content/uploads/2014/01/English-OTIPM-handout.pdf. Reprinted with permission.

INTRODUCTION

As occupational therapists, when we start working with a client, the first thing we do is find out about their current situation and priority areas (creating an *occupational profile*, as described in Chapter 4). We do this through talking with people, and observing them in their environment. Therefore, the three OTIPM steps discussed in this chapter occur *simultaneously*. Together, they are a vital starting point to any occupational therapy process.

STEP 1: "DEVELOP THERAPEUTIC RAPPORT AND WORKING COLLABORATIVELY WITH THE CLIENT"

You will be able to achieve a great deal more if clients and your colleagues in the team or therapy setting trust in your suggestions and feel comfortable talking to you about their concerns. To do this you need to "Develop therapeutic rapport and work collaboratively with the client(s)." This is one of the *most important* aspects to your placement.

Developing these relationships is a long-term process and something which you need to *continuously work on*. It is not something that you will finish in one step of the occupational therapy process. The ongoing nature of developing rapport and collaborative relationships is indicated by the arrows throughout the whole OTIPM flow diagram (Figure 6.1).

Developing therapeutic rapport and working collaboratively with others involves *being available, visible, approachable* and *helpful*. You may start your interactions by introducing yourself, explaining your role and why you are involved with this service and/or person (as described in Chapter 5). When developing rapport, you may find that you do not talk about occupational therapy much at all, but instead have a general conversation to get to know who the person is and share a little about yourself.

Adopt a positive attitude and always assume that the person you are developing rapport with has many skills, competencies, beliefs, values, commitments and abilities. You want to find out what these are; ask the person questions about things they enjoy, are good at, beliefs they might hold, things that are important to them and commitments they might have in their life. These have the added benefit of ultimately being able to inform your occupational therapy practice as well as demonstrate that you are interested in the person you are speaking to, and hold a positive view about them. Curiosity about people, and a willingness to ask questions, are important skills for an occupational therapist. Some further ideas about this process may be considered from *narrative and interactive reasoning* perspectives (Turpin and Copley, 2017; Schell and Schell, 2008), which are described in more detail in Chapters 7 and 11.

Vitally important to this process is your *body language*, which signals your approachability and interest in the person, and can convey a sense of trust. Maintaining appropriate eye contact, and subtly mirroring the person's body language can also help place the person at ease and increase their sense of being listened to, and their trust in you. Also, be conscious of where you are focusing your attention. You can be easily diverted (e.g. by using a mobile phone or speaking with colleagues) and being distracted can demonstrate a lack of interest in the person.

You will have a range of reasons to make connections with people during your placement. You may need to discuss with people what experiences they have had previously with occupational therapists. This might impact on the expectations they have for what you do in the placement. For example, if a teacher has had experiences of an occupational therapist taking a child out of his/her classroom to do a programme of activities, you may need to spend time with him/her explaining that your approach will be supporting children do their occupations within the classroom. Understanding expectations can help you determine how best to communicate your initial observations, plans and progress as well as how often you might need to speak, email or formally meet with people.

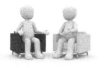

ACTIVITY
....

Table 6.1 offers suggestions for how you might develop rapport and collaborative relationships when in a school context. Consider these suggestions and then develop at least five ways in which you could develop rapport within your own placement context. Use these ideas as a basis for discussion with a peer and in your supervision.

Table 6.1 Strategies for developing rapport in a school context

Ask the class teacher how he/she would like the children to address you.

Assist if children are struggling or help with the set up or clearing up of equipment and materials. Be helpful, but you need to balance this with not appearing to take on the role of a teaching assistant.

Provide appropriate feedback after each classroom observation. Think about how you might feel if someone was observing your practice and then walked out straight after the session without making any comment.

Find time to talk with teachers. You may need to 'catch' them at times such as when the children are in assembly, or if you are helping to set up the classroom for the next activity.

Eat your lunch and take your breaks in the staff room with the teachers. Being a familiar person around the school is important.

Find out as much as you can about the education curriculum. Acknowledge the teacher's expertise by seeking his/her advice and guidance.

STEPS 2 AND 3: "ESTABLISH CLIENT-CENTRED PERFORMANCE CONTEXT," AND "IDENTIFY RESOURCES AND LIMITATIONS WITHIN CLIENT-CENTRED PERFORMANCE CONTEXT"

At the same time as we are developing therapeutic relationships, we are also focused on trying to "Establish the client-centred performance context." This means we want to find out about the person or people with whom we will be working. We want to know what is important for that person, how the person feels able to do his/her occupations and how satisfied the person is with fulfilling life roles. We want to know where the person carries out the occupations he/she wants to, needs to or is expected to do. We also want to find out about a person's interests and motivations, his/her age and background (Fisher, 2009).

In gathering this information, we are starting to develop an occupational profile and a picture of some of the "Resources and limitations within the client-centred performance context." This could be people who are supportive, adaptations in the environment, policy direction, availability of funding or opportunities for change (Fisher, 2009).

WHO IS THE CLIENT?

When we think about who it is we are working with, rarely are we just thinking of one person. We all exist in social groups such as in a family, with teachers and classmates in a school, in a residential facility with staff members and other residents, or in a workplace with colleagues. Often when a person is challenged in doing his/her occupations, it also impacts on, and is impacted by, others. Therefore, we need to consider not just the person who has challenges in his/her own occupational performance, but also the needs of those around that person. Fisher (2009, p. 3) calls this group the 'client constellation'.

For example, on placement you may be working with a child who has cerebral palsy who wants to write a story in class. You would need to consider the needs of the child, but also those of the teacher, parents and classmates. If you were working in a hospital supporting people to return home after surgery, you would need to consider the people, the carers (paid or unpaid) of the people at home, and the views of medical and nursing staff on the ward. At times, you may also be considering the needs of a group of people who may have similar issues but are otherwise unrelated. For example, you might be working with a group of wheelchair users to access public transport, or you could be working with local government supporting the implementation of a childhood obesity strategy.

The key point when thinking about 'who is the client?' is to identify who is crucial in the situation. This is so you can consider the needs of all relevant people and negotiate the priority areas for your involvement, which could initially focus on the occupations of others in a situation.

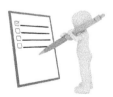

ACTIVITY
....

Make a list of the people whom you encounter in the placement. Think about who the client is – a person, a group, a community or a population. Consider who is surrounding that client that you may also need to involve. Use this as a discussion point with your peer and in supervision.

FINDING OUT WHO TO CONTACT

To understand the placement setting you will need to spend time with the staff members and clients. In your first one to two weeks, discuss and develop your timetable with your educator and plan to observe in several different locations (and different occupations) in the setting.

ACTIVITY

Create a way to record who you need to liaise with and keep informed of your progress (you could use the examples in Table 6.2 to create a template). Clarify the best method for contacting people such as in meetings, emails or informal catch-ups.

Table 6.2 Contact sheet example

Name: Austin David | **Position:** On-site supervisor/Manager
Phone number: 1234 5678 | **Email:** austin.david@carehome.com
Preferred contact method: Email or face-to-face
Level of contact required: Weekly updates during supervision, email other times, informal contact fine if there are questions.

Name: Lucy Cook | **Position:** Long-arm supervisor/lecturer
Phone number: 9876 6543 | **Email:** Lucy.cook@university.com
Preferred contact method: Email, telephone, face-to-face
Level of contact required: Weekly supervision, email as needed, telephone if arranged

FINDING OUT ABOUT THE PLACEMENT ENVIRONMENT

Observing what happens in the placement setting will help you identify supports and potential barriers to facilitating occupation (i.e. "Identifying resources and limitations within the client-centred performance context").

When you are planning your timetable of observations, think about how you might introduce yourself, explain what you are looking at and how you will discuss your findings with those involved. For example, if you are observing a nurse run a group in an acute mental health setting, you could say:

"I am an occupational therapy student and I would like to see how you run your group. This is part of my induction to the setting to help me understand what people do here and how they do it.

I'll be using a form to help me structure what I am looking at so that I can begin to relate what I am seeing back to occupational therapy. My aim is to help support people to do their occupations.

The areas I will be specifically looking at include things like what the group does, how long they spend on activities, how the room's space and furniture might affect the group and how people interact with each other. I might make some notes to help me and I wondered if that was OK with you?

I am also keen to hear your thoughts about the group. It would be great to arrange a time to talk together, perhaps after I have had a chance to reflect on things. Would that be possible?"

Observations can take many forms. If you do not already have a way of structuring your observations (from your university or the placement setting's existing frameworks), you could use the general context observation sheet (Table 6.3, and downloadable from website www.routledge.com/9781138238480).

Table 6.3 General observations sheet

Setting (e.g. dining hall, kitchen, bedroom):
Date/time:
People present:

Culture

What is the setting atmosphere and expectations?
How do client(s), staff and significant others relate to each other?

Social

How many people are generally in the context?
When are there opportunities for playing and socialising?
What are the expected social norms and routines (e.g. classroom rules, expectations of independence)?

Temporal

Is the setting routine structured or unstructured?
What is this order of events and how long is each activity?
How do the clients know about the routine?
Does the routine change from day to day? If so, how do the clients know about these changes?
Are there set routines (e.g. mealtimes, going to the toilet, sleep etc.)?

Virtual

How often are computers/tablets/phones/technology used?
Does anybody use augmentative communication equipment?
How comfortable do you think the staff and clients are using computers and other technology?

(Continued)

Table 6.3 (Continued)

Physical

Where do the clients store their personal belongings? Is this accessible?

Are the buildings accessible for a wheelchair user or someone with restricted mobility?

Are the toilets and sinks accessible to all clients?

Is the space adequate (consider the space for working, sitting, socialising, moving around the environment, eating lunch etc.)?

What are the textures of the materials, furniture and carpet?

What is the usual noise level in this space?

What is the lighting like in this space? Is there any glare?

Are there visual distractions, i.e. notice boards, open shelves, decorations?

Are there movement opportunities for the clients? If so, how frequently?

What is the temperature of the space?

Draw a scale diagram (or take a photo if you have permission) of the physical environment. Include all of the permanent structures (doors, windows, steps, equipment etc.), moveable structures (chairs, tables, shelves etc.) and label how the clients move around the space.

Any other comments?

Source: Dancza and Volkert (2018). Downloadable at www.routledge.com/9781138238480. Adapted from Hanft and Shepherd (2008, pp. 234–236).

These general observations will give you an overview of where the clients are performing their occupations, and perhaps an idea of where clients may need support to further enable their participation.

REPORTING BACK ON YOUR OBSERVATIONS

The purpose of the general context observation is to develop your own understanding of the setting. You may use this information to supplement the assessment you complete later in the occupational therapy process.

After the observation, your client(s) and those in the setting are likely to want some feedback. This can be daunting for students as you often need time and discussion with your educator to consolidate what you saw and clarify what is important to share. Finding the balance of sharing some brief information which you are confident about at this early stage can help develop relationships. This could include a few positives about your observations and a question about an aspect that you would like to know more about. For example, if you were speaking with the nurse following the observation of a group, you could say:

> "Thank you, Kaaren, for allowing me to observe the group. I found it interesting how you included all participants and managed the situation when one person was speaking a lot. I wanted to know a bit more about why you directed the group to focus on their experiences of their symptoms. I will be discussing some of my thoughts with my educator, but could we arrange to meet sometime to talk about it more?"

Remember that if you mention that you will follow something up then it is important to do so – *don't promise things you don't deliver!*

When you have time to go through your observation in more detail, you will need to consider which information is meaningful for the staff members and clients, rather than just presenting your completed general observation sheet notes. You can discuss this further with your educator, but as an opening you could say something like:

> "Thank you for allowing me in your classroom, I found it really valuable observing John. I noticed that he looks around the classroom a lot and does not always focus on his work. Is this something which you have noticed as well? What do you think is happening when he does this?
>
> What I observed was John looking over to the group of children at the next table who were chatting about the work they were doing. I also noticed that John's chair was bumped frequently as children moved past him to get to their drawers. Is this something you have noticed?"

The things you can provide feedback on at this stage are still general as you have not yet prioritised what is important and completed a detailed occupational performance analysis (see Chapters 7 and 8). If there are a few things, however, which could easily be changed at this stage (such as slightly moving the table so John's chair isn't bumped), then it may help those in the service setting see that you are trying to be useful and it could support the development of your therapeutic relationships.

REFLECTION ON THE FIRST WEEK OF PLACEMENT

By the end of the first week you will find that you have learnt a lot about the placement setting, but there are probably more questions than answers for you at this stage. Reflection can help you make sense of what is happening. Depending on how you like to reflect, try one of the following reflection techniques:

– Find an image which represents how you are feeling about your placement now. Attach the image and explain in a few sentences what it represents. Then share this with your student peer.

or

– Consider the following questions either on your own or through a discussion with your student peer.
  – Think about your own skills: what are you feeling confident about now?
  – What are you unsure of and would like to find out more about?
  – From your university studies, what do you think you need to revise/look again at?

CHAPTER SUMMARY

In this chapter, we have looked at the three initial phases of the OTIPM (Fisher, 2009), encompassing the first one to two weeks of a placement. Developing rapport and working collaboratively will take time, but it is vital for anything you wish to do. Being seen in the placement context, talking with people and providing some initial feedback about what you're doing are helpful ways for you to get to know the placement setting and for them to get to know you. Observing in a range of contexts and different occupations is a helpful way for you to understand the placement setting and get to know the staff members and clients. We presented a format for these observations so that you are focused on relevant aspects within the environment. The next chapter will explore how to gather more specific information about the priorities of occupational performance for people you will be working with.

REFERENCES

Fisher AG (2009) *Occupational therapy intervention process model: A model for planning and implementing top-down, client centred, and occupation-based interventions*. Fort Collins, CO: Three Star Press.

Hanft BE, Shepherd J, eds (2008) *Collaborating for student success: A guide for school-based occupational therapy*. Bethesda, MD: American Occupational Therapy Association Press.

Schell BAB, Schell JW, eds (2008) *Clinical and professional reasoning in occupational therapy*. Philadelphia, PA: Walters Kluwer/Lippincott, Williams & Wilkins.

Turpin MJ, Copley JA, (2018) 'Interactive reasoning'. In BAB Schell, JW Schell (Eds.), *Clinical and professional reasoning in occupational therapy*, 2nd ed. Philadelphia, PA: Wolters Kluwer/Lippincott, Williams & Wilkins, pp. 245–260.

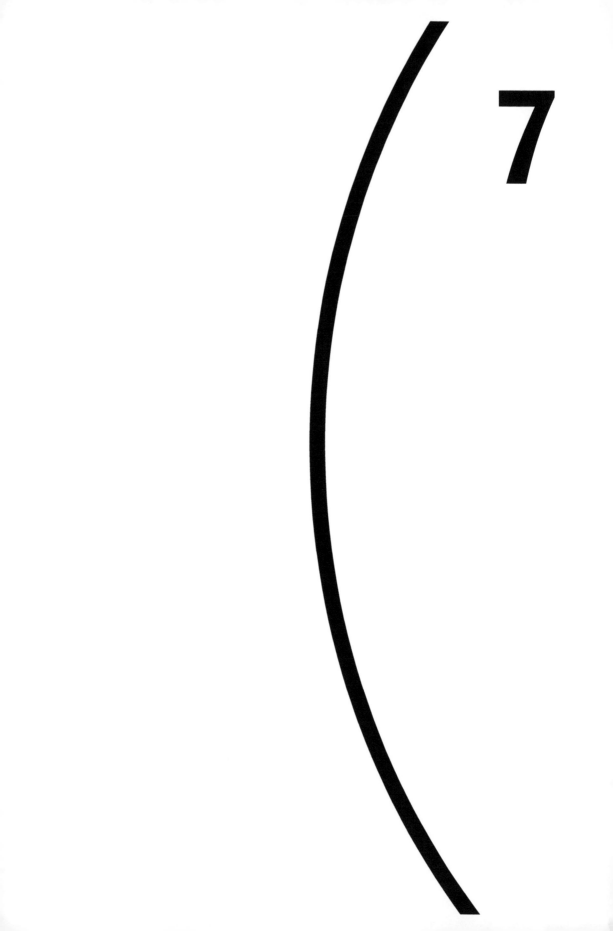

7

CHAPTER 7
IDENTIFYING CLIENT'S REPORTED AND PRIORITIZED STRENGTHS AND PROBLEMS OF OCCUPATIONAL PERFORMANCE
Karina Dancza and Jodie Copley

INTENDED CHAPTER OUTCOMES

By the end of this chapter, readers will have an overview of:

- Influences on the prioritisation of clients' occupational needs in role-established and role-emerging placements
- Strategies to guide the prioritisation process
- How interactive reasoning can be used to understand and prioritise clients' occupational needs

STAGE IN THE OTIPM

As we presented in Chapter 6, your work as a student occupational therapist is informed by practice models such as the Occupational Therapy Intervention Process Model (OTIPM; Fisher, 2009). In this chapter, we are focusing on the prioritisation stage of a client's occupational performance strengths and challenges. Please take a few moments to revisit the OTIPM flow diagram (Figure 7.1), to familiarise yourself with where we are in the process.

INTRODUCTION

This chapter describes the skills and practices that may assist you to "Identify client's reported and prioritized strengths and problems of occupational performance." You will have some ideas from your own observations and initial discussions with the staff members and clients, but you will probably need to gather some more specific information to clarify expectations and ensure you have support from all relevant people involved with the client(s).

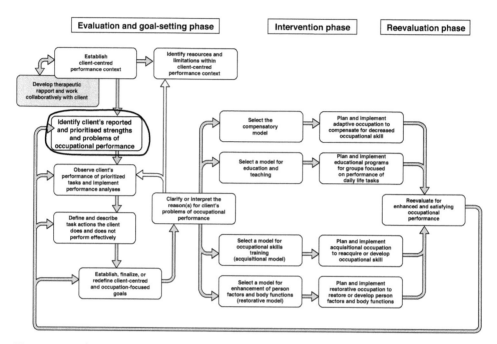

Figure 7.1 Schematic representation of the steps in the OTIPM: Identify client's reported and prioritized strengths and problems of occupational performance

Adapted from Fisher (2009). Available: www.innovativeotsolutions.com/content/wp-content/uploads/2014/01/English-OTIPM-handout.pdf. Reprinted with permission.

There can be different influences on how this process occurs in role-established placements compared with role-emerging placements. These two situations, therefore, will be introduced separately. However, some practices could be applied to role-emerging, role-established or project placements.

ROLE-ESTABLISHED PLACEMENTS

When you begin a role-established placement, you are coming into an organisation with its own internal policies and procedures which, together with your educator's intentions to introduce you to certain aspects of practice, will determine which clients you will see. In some organisations, these policies also dictate how often and how long you will be involved.

For example, in an inpatient stroke unit, hospital policy (which may be influenced by national stroke guidelines and research evidence) may dictate that all patients are seen daily during the first two months of rehabilitation. At a community developmental service for children, service delivery policies may specify that after initial intake, all families are offered a block of eight therapy sessions. These parameters determine, to a large extent, your caseload whilst on placement.

In addition to organisational policies, the understood roles and expectations of the occupational therapist (your educator) from his/her interdisciplinary team members and the organisation further determines your focus. For example, in one organisation, the occupational therapy role might emphasise upper limb and cognitive rehabilitation, whilst in another service, the focus is on self-management in the community. These differences shape the extent to which, firstly, your role is centred on occupation, and secondly, you can prioritise which occupational needs are dealt with.

ACTIVITY

Investigate and summarise at least two national policies and two local/setting policies or priorities which might have an impact on the work you do with clients in this setting. Use these summaries as discussion points with your peer (if available) and your educator.

Given the range of influences on your work, it is important that you have discussions with your educator about how you will prioritise clients' occupational needs. It is most likely that within a role-established setting, the clients you will work with are already referred for occupational therapy. However, you will still need to determine with the client, family and significant others (the client constellation as described in Chapter 6) which occupations are important and should be the focus for your involvement. There may be opportunities for you to look at a wider range of occupations or work on projects which extend the role your educator has with a few clients, as you are an additional person in the setting.

ROLE-EMERGING PLACEMENTS

Role-emerging placements (and some project placements) are different in that they do not have the same established occupational therapy processes or understanding of the role of the occupational therapist as do role-established placements. However, like role-established placements, they do have their own policy context and priorities for service delivery of which you need to be aware.

When you enter a role-emerging placement, you will need to gain a general understanding of the placement setting (as explored in Chapter 6) and its priority areas. You will need to prioritise for yourself (with your on-site and long-arm supervisors) who to work with and what to work on. You need to be mindful that you only have a limited time on placement in which to get to know the setting, plan and implement interventions.

Prioritisation is a challenging skill. Even experienced occupational therapists can struggle with this task. For you, with intermittent guidance available on a day-to-day basis, valuable time can be wasted by attempting to take on too many projects or tasks which are not going to be beneficial to your learning. In the following sections we outline some practical guidance for helping you determine priority areas. We will then explore how you will need to use your interactive reasoning skills (Turpin and Copley, 2017) to successfully prioritise in partnership with your client(s). Prioritisation is a skill you will need to develop during role-established, role-emerging or project placements.

CONSIDERING CULTURE AND DIFFERENCE

As occupational therapists, we work with people of all ages and from all backgrounds. We therefore need to work sensitively and responsively with those who differ from our own experiences. Sometimes this is referred to as being 'culturally capable' or 'culturally competent' (Grant, Parry and Guerin, 2013). Culture, in its broadest sense, may be considered to encompass age, sexuality, religion, gender, class and belief systems as well as ethnicity (Nelson, McLaren, Lewis and Iwama, 2017). It is important to be aware of our own beliefs and values. We should actively seek to find out about the cultures of people with whom we work, rather than make assumptions based on our previous personal experience (or internet searches!).

We need to incorporate the priorities, needs and wishes of our client(s) into the occupational therapy process. At times, these may differ from our own notions. For example, the belief that it is important to complete self-care independently is a feature of Western culture, but in many Eastern cultures this would not be a priority in someone's rehabilitation after a stroke. The client may prefer to work on other aspects of his/her occupational life, and family members may wish to incorporate the self-care of the client into their own occupational roles. Another example of how our beliefs can influence our actions as a therapist might be a reluctance to discuss and address issues with an older person's sex life, based on the incorrect assumption that older people do not have an active sex life.

ACTIVITY

1   If you are working with someone from a different background/culture who you want to find out more about, ask to spend some time with them. Questions that you might wish to ask include:
    –   What language do you speak most often?
    –   What kinds of foods are cooked/eaten in your culture/from your background?

- Are there different roles for men/women/children in your culture?
- Is it important for you to do things by yourself or with support from others (such as self-care, meal preparation, budgeting)?
- Who do you go to for advice?
- What thing(s) would you like to share with me about your culture/background?

2   In some settings, there may be a member of staff or volunteer who can help you understand specific cultural groups. Ask your educator for guidance as to who you could approach.

3   You may also have an opportunity to work with an interpreter or telephone interpreting service. This is an excellent opportunity to extend your skills and gain a greater understanding of your client. Talk to the interpreter and your educator about the communication protocols for successfully working with this service.

4   For more information on cultural influences and occupation-centred practice, please see Nelson et al. (2017).

IDENTIFYING PRIORITY AREAS: A STEP-BY-STEP GUIDE

In role-established, role-emerging or project placements, you will need to find out from key stakeholders in the setting (such as staff members and clients) what they see as priorities for your involvement. In role-emerging settings, you may find, however, that they do not readily identify what the occupational therapy priorities might be, as they are unsure of what occupational therapy can provide. People may also make suggestions about what they think you can offer (or what has historically been offered), without knowing the full scope of the occupational therapy role. You may need to have some ideas to share to begin the conversation, but also take the time needed for people to think about and discuss what is important to them.

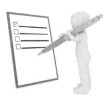

ACTIVITY
....

Table 7.1 gives some examples of priority areas which came up for a student in a role-emerging placement in a primary school in the United Kingdom. From your observations and discussions in your setting, list some ideas for your possible involvement. Use this list as a discussion point with your peer (if available) and your educator.

Table 7.1 Examples of priority areas for occupational therapy student involvement

Possible priority areas	Person who identified the area
Children in the year 1 class not being able to see the whiteboard when in their seats	Occupational therapy student
The lack of independence of children when eating breakfast during Breakfast Club	Head teacher
The time taken for children to settle into class after break time	Teacher
The anxiety and performance of secondary school students when completing a year 9 maths practice exam	Students

GATHERING INFORMATION TO DETERMINE PRIORITY AREAS

The questions you ask and how you gather information will depend on your client group and setting. Remember that your domain of concern is the *occupations* of the people in the setting, so try to keep conversations focused. Look back at the occupations you listed in Chapter 5 which may be relevant to your client group.

Asking open-ended questions can promote discussion about priority areas. You may speak with people on a one-to-one basis, talk to a group in a meeting or develop a questionnaire. Developing a questionnaire can help if people are not able to give you time to meet face-to-face, if there are many people whose opinion you need to canvas, or if you wish to have some data which justifies your reasoning processes. The activity which follows provides some examples of questions you could use. Table 7.2 provides an example of a questionnaire developed by students for teachers during a school-based role-emerging placement. The scales were also used as an outcome measure following the interventions.

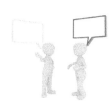

ACTIVITY

Look through these example questions (adapted from Hasselbusch and Dunford, 2011, p. 9). Make a list of your own questions which are relevant for your client group and setting.

1   Can you tell me about a typical day?
2   What things about the day do you/does *[name of client]* enjoy or like?
3   What activities do you/does *[name of client]* find tricky or struggle with?
4   Are there any times during the day which are more difficult for you/the client(s)? For example:
   –   Mealtimes
   –   Transitioning between activities

- Talking with others
- Moving around
- Particular activities
- Using the toilet

5 To follow up these areas you could ask:
  - Can you tell me a bit more about what happens [during the activity]?
  - [to staff members] Is it only one client, or do a few clients find this challenging?
  - What have you tried before which has helped or not helped?
  - How do you expect this activity to be done?

6 If you came in to the setting tomorrow and things had really improved, what would you notice? What would be different? What might the client/family members/other staff say is different?

7 Imagine we are sitting here talking in [three months / six months/ one year] from now. What would you like/[name of client] to be able to do?

Table 7.2 Priority questionnaire for teachers

School participation questionnaire for teachers

Name of child/class:

Date:

Person completing the form:

Doing schoolwork
Being in the classroom
Undertaking school routines
Looking after oneself
Organising oneself
Moving around the school
Socialising and leisure

Please circle the areas of primary concern

Specify which two activities you would like to focus on within the primary area(s) of concern

1.
2.

1 2 3 4 5
1 2 3 4 5

Rate how satisfied you are currently with how the activity is being undertaken, where 1 is not at all satisfied and 5 is extremely satisfied

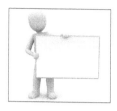

EDUCATOR EXAMPLES HERE: QUESTIONS
FOR ESTABLISHING PRIORITIES

— Ask your educator if there are additional questions you could ask clients or staff
  members. You could also refer back to your university learning about interviewing.

DETERMINING PRIORITIES: QUESTIONS FOR CHILDREN AND VULNERABLE ADULTS

Finding out what is important for clients may not always be as straightforward as asking
them during a formal interview. When you are working with children, vulnerable adults
or people with different communication needs, you will need to check with your educator
about the best way to gather the clients' opinions. For example, when working in a school
setting or residential care facility, you could gather the opinions of children or older adults
in general conversation while you are interacting with them in an activity. The types of
questions and way you ask them also requires consideration. There may also be different
requirements for gaining consent.

Hanft and Shepherd (2008, p. 39) suggested the following questions, which may offer a
starting point for developing your own questions for children. You might also adapt these
questions for other vulnerable client groups. Think about the occupations the client needs
to do, for example in his/her role as student.

— What do you like best about school/work setting/care home?
— What is easy for you/what are you good at?
— What don't you like to do?
— What is hard for you?
— What is your favourite part of the day?
— If you could change one thing, what would it be?

Keep your language clear and simple. Use visual prompts if appropriate (e.g. card
sorts, goal-setting tools) and allow the person time to respond to your question
(pauses in conversation are fine!). Sometimes it might be useful to silently count to
ten after you have asked a question to give time for the person to process the question
and construct a response. If the person does not respond, you could repeat your
question, rephrase your question or use a visual prompt. Remember if you ask the
question again using different words you need to allow time for the person to process
this new question.

Consider the environment (noise level, lighting, distractions) and time of day when
you are asking questions. Think of novel ways to gather opinions, such as writing ideas
on pieces of paper and sticking them up on the wall. *Taking photos* is a useful way of

recording not only ideas, but also the environment where the occupations are performed. This is useful if you are hoping to make changes to the environment. Ensure you have permission to take photos and be careful about including clients or staff members in any images unless you have permission.

Some students on placement have used the *Kawa River metaphor* (Iwama, 2006) to gain the opinions of clients about their occupational performance strengths and challenges. It may be that clients draw and label their own river, or use pre-cut pieces to show their river. See Iwama (2006) or www.kawamodel.com for further ideas.

Some clients who experience challenges communicating may need different strategies. Parents, staff members and other professionals in the setting can offer ideas for gaining the perspectives of the client. A useful text to find out more about this is Powrie and Hemsley (2015) and this is discussed in relation to goal setting in Chapter 10.

PRIORITISING IS MORE COMPLEX THAN ASKING QUESTIONS

USING INTERACTIVE REASONING TO ESTABLISH OCCUPATIONAL PRIORITIES – ADVICE FOR STUDENTS

Finding out what people want is a complex process as every situation is different. You need to ask the 'right' questions at the 'right' time and respond appropriately to the person with whom you are interacting. To successfully establish priority areas that are meaningful to clients and significant others in their lives, occupational therapists use a process called 'interactive reasoning'. Building skills in interactive reasoning supports you to foster relationships (as described in Chapter 5 when developing rapport with clients). It enables you to develop an understanding of the person and his/her life context, and in partnership, shape a meaningful vision of the future (Turpin and Copley, 2017).

Interactive reasoning is related to therapeutic use of self (Taylor, 2014) and requires tailoring one's interpersonal skills (body position, gestures, facial expressions, voice, use of humour, use of conversation, etc.) in a skilled manner to establish a connection with clients. This allows in-depth information gathering of a client's occupational profile and what is important to them (Turpin and Copley, 2017).

To decide which priorities may be worth pursuing through intervention, you must reason *in the moment*. This is where you process information provided by the client and interview in a responsive way, clarifying and probing further until a vivid picture is established (Turpin and Copley, 2017). Simultaneously, you apply your own expertise to think about what outcomes might be possible for this person, given his/her current situation, abilities and resources, as well as what interventions are available and how they might respond to these (Copley, Turpin, Brosnan and Nelson, 2008).

With all this information in mind, a process of negotiating occurs. This is where you begin with the client's goals and offer information to the client and significant others about what types of therapy targets might be realistic to aim for that move the client closer to his/her goals (Copley et al., 2008). Essentially, you are balancing the role of information seeker and expert consultant – in other words, balancing actively listening to the client's concerns and drawing on his/her knowledge with sharing expertise to assist his/her situation. This information will be used in Chapter 8 to frame your observational assessment and Chapter 10 when you refine the goals.

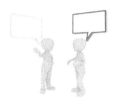

ACTIVITY
....

1   Think about a conversation you had with a client and reflect on what you said and did. How did you know that you had the right information?
2   If possible, observe your educator and discuss afterwards how he/she structured an interaction, what made them ask certain questions, why he/she probed further on a point, what they noticed about the client's responses, etc.

USING INTERACTIVE REASONING TO ESTABLISH OCCUPATIONAL PRIORITIES – A NOTE FOR EDUCATORS

As educators, it is important that we explicitly guide students to develop their reasoning skills and not expect students to 'magically' understand through experience alone. Demonstrating your own reasoning to students is a useful strategy. In teaching students the complex skill of interactive reasoning, helpful processes and tools may include:

–   Ensuring that students use the occupational therapy model favoured by your organisation, so that they have a framework to comprehensively explore relevant aspects of the clients' occupational roles and performance. Demonstrating how it might integrate with the OTIPM is useful if students are following the structure of this book.
–   Creating, or helping students create, a flexible interviewing tool that allows them to tailor their questions to each client and their individual context and be responsive to the answers provided, probing and clarifying as needed to form a clear occupational picture. The checklists and closed-ended interview tools sometimes used in practice settings can be limited in encouraging clients to tell their occupational narrative in sufficient detail to guide decisions about priorities for therapy.
–   Developing reasoning tools can help students articulate their decision making and how information about the client has led to the priorities chosen. Tools could include assessment forms, decision trees or concept maps that illustrate what factors about the client, his/her context, the therapist and the organisation have been considered in making these decisions (see also Chapter 11 for further examples).

- Encouraging students to ask you questions about why you made a decision, what you noticed about how the person reacted, why you asked another question, etc. Students benefit from observing how you manage uncertainty and unpredictable responses when interacting with clients.

SUMMARISING YOUR PRIORITY AREAS

Interactive reasoning focuses on the conversations you have with clients. Once you feel that you have fully explored the priority areas with the client, take a moment to summarise them so that the client can clarify his/her perspectives if needed and you will have a clear picture of what he/she sees as important. This will help you determine what you will assess further in the next chapter and stage of the OTIPM.

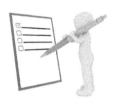

ACTIVITY

After gathering the information from the service setting, staff members and clients, revisit your earlier brainstorm about your priority areas and make a new list of ones you wish to pursue (there should be two or three maximum at this stage).

SIX THINKING HATS TO REFLECT ON THE SUITABILITY
OF YOUR PRIORITIES

You have already given considerable effort to the development of your priority areas. Just to be sure you have considered all relevant aspects, you could use a reflective tool. The Six Thinking Hats (De Bono, 1985) activity encourages you to think about a priority area from six different perspectives, each labelled with a different coloured hat. You could use this for self-reflection, or as prompt questions for a discussion with your peer or educator. This technique could also be useful during other parts of your occupational therapy process (such as intervention planning in Chapter 12).

ACTIVITY

Take a few minutes to write something for each hat in Table 7.3. You can then use this as a basis to discuss your priority areas with your educator.

Table 7.3 Six Thinking Hats activity

White Hat – facts, information, data, research needed

What information is available?

What more do you need?

What information is missing?

Red Hat – feelings, hunches, emotions, intuition

What are your feelings about ___?

What does your intuition tell you?

No justification is required.

Black Hat – caution, risks, judgement

What could be possible problems?

What should you be cautious of?

What are the risks?

Green Hat – creativity, new ideas, brainstorming, predicting

What are the alternatives and possibilities?

How can we overcome our Black Hat difficulties?

What are other ways to do this?

Blue Hat – thinking about thinking, metacognition, summarizing

How will you summarise your idea for:

Your long-arm supervisor?

Your on-site supervisor?

The client(s)?

Yellow Hat – benefits, value, strengths

What are the benefits?

What did you like about . . .

How will this help?

What is the potential?

CHAPTER SUMMARY

This chapter explored the differences between role-established and role-emerging placements when prioritising occupational therapy involvement. We presented a step-by-step guide to the prioritisation process which could be used in role-established, role-emerging or project placements. This process is, however, more complicated than allowed for in a step-by-step guide. Interactive reasoning is required in the to-and-fro exchanges with clients to successfully prioritise occupational strengths and needs.

REFERENCES

Copley J, Turpin M, Brosnan J, Nelson A (2008) 'Reasoning processes used to individualise intervention decisions for people with upper limb hypertonicity'. *Disability and Rehabilitation*, *30*(19), 1486–1498.

De Bono E (1985) *Six Thinking Hats: An essential approach to business management.* London, UK: Little, Brown and Company.

Fisher AG (2009) *Occupational therapy intervention process model: A model for planning and implementing top-down, client centred, and occupation-based interventions.* Fort Collins, CO: Three Star Press.

Grant J, Parry Y, Guerin P (2013) 'An investigation of culturally competent terminology in healthcare policy finds ambiguity and lack of definition'. *Australian and New Zealand Journal of Public Health*, *37*(3), 250–256.

Hanft BE, Shepherd J, eds (2008) *Collaborating for student success: A guide for school-based occupational therapy.* Bethesda, MD: American Occupational Therapy Association Press.

Hasselbusch A, Dunford C (2011) 'Use of the Canadian Occupational Performance Measure in school-based occupational therapy'. *Children, Young People & Families Occupational Therapy Journal*, *15*(2), 5–12.

Iwama MK (2006) *The Kawa model: Culturally relevant occupational therapy.* Edinburgh: Churchill Livingstone.

Nelson A, McLaren C, Lewis T, Iwama MK (2017) 'Cultural influences and occupation-centred practice with children and families'. In: S Rodger, A Kennedy-Behr, eds, *Occupation-centred practice with children: A practical guide for occupational therapists.* 2nd edn. West Sussex, UK: Wiley-Blackwell, pp. 73–90.

Powrie B, Hemsley B (2015) 'Goal identification when communication is a challenge'. In: A Poulsen, J Ziviani, M Cuskelly, eds, *Goal setting and motivation in therapy: Engaging children and parents.* London: Jessica Kingsley Publishers, pp. 131–142.

Taylor RR (2014) 'Therapeutic relationship and client collaboration'. In: BAB Schell, G Gillen, ME Scaffa, eds, *Willard & Spackman's occupational therapy.* 12th edn. Philadelphia, PA: Lippincott Williams & Wilkins, pp. 425–436.

Turpin MJ, Copley JA, (2018) 'Interactive reasoning'. In BAB Schell, JW Schell (Eds.), *Clinical and professional reasoning in occupational therapy*, 2nd ed. Philadelphia, PA: Wolters Kluwer/Lippincott, Williams & Wilkins, pp. 245–260.

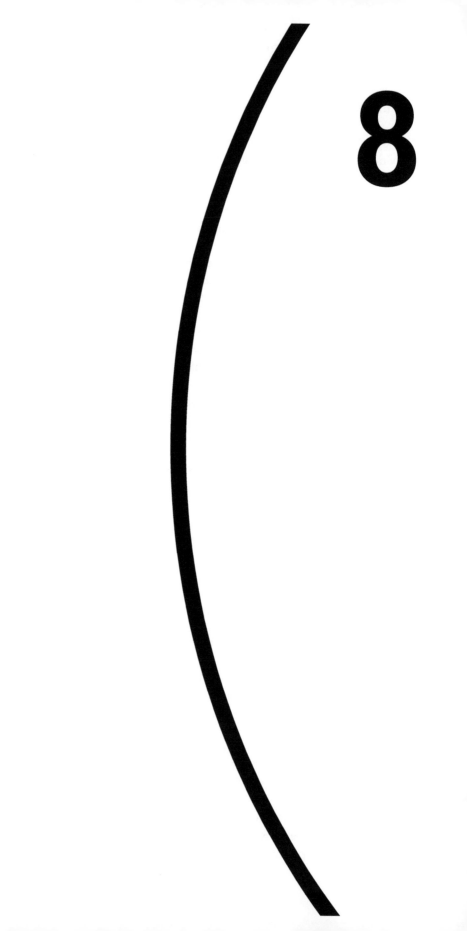

8

OBSERVING CLIENT'S PERFORMANCE OF PRIORITISED TASKS AND IMPLEMENTING PERFORMANCE ANALYSIS

Sue Mesa, Karina Dancza and Jeannette Head

INTENDED CHAPTER OUTCOMES

By the end of this chapter, readers will have an overview of:

- How planning for outcome measurement begins during assessment
- What to consider when preparing for an observational assessment
- How to practically carry out an observational assessment using an occupational performance analysis
- Advice for educators to support students undertaking assessments

STAGE IN THE OTIPM

From the prioritisation of occupational performance strengths and needs in Chapter 7, the next stage in the Occupational Therapy Intervention Process Model (OTIPM; Fisher, 2009) is to undertake an observational assessment. This is shown in the OTIPM flow diagram (Figure 8.1). Please take a few minutes to familiarise where you are in the occupational therapy process in preparation for your detailed assessment outlined in this chapter.

INTRODUCTION

Detailed assessment in the OTIPM is referred to as "Observe the client's performance of prioritised tasks and implement a performance analysis." Observing the person and completing an *occupational performance analysis* will enable you to gain a thorough understanding of how they carry out the occupation. It will highlight how the person is currently doing his/her occupations and where improvements might be made (considering the person–environment–occupation interplay). This should help you to plan appropriate interventions and later, enable you to measure the outcomes of your interventions.

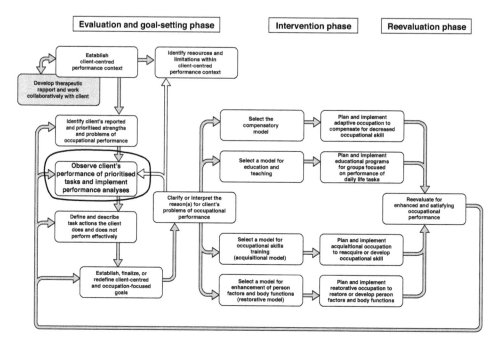

Figure 8.1 Schematic representation of the steps in the OTIPM: Observe client's performance of prioritized tasks and implement performance analysis

Adapted from Fisher (2009). Available: www.innovativeotsolutions.com/content/wp-content/uploads/2014/01/English-OTIPM-handout.pdf. Reprinted with permission.

There are assessment methods which you can use to gather relevant information to plan intervention. As we wish to present a coherent way to carry out the occupational therapy process using the OTIPM, this chapter outlines how you might prepare and carry out an observational assessment, using activity and occupational performance analysis as your key tools (see the templates in Chapter 4). We do, however, acknowledge that this may not always be possible and we discuss what you might do in these situations later in the chapter. We also encourage you to think about gathering information now that you can use to evaluate the impact of your interventions in later stages of the OTIPM.

HOW ACTIVITY ANALYSIS FITS INTO THE OCCUPATIONAL THERAPY PROCESS

Careful analysis of a person doing a priority occupation is one of the cornerstones of occupational therapy. Having completed an *occupational profile* (Chapter 6), and developed occupational priorities with the client (Chapter 7), you will have a plan of what you will observe.

While this is not a separate step in the OTIPM, completing an *activity analysis* will support your understanding of the components of the prioritised activity. For the novice practitioner, it is recommended that you use a set structure, such as the template in Chapter 4. As noted by Chard and Mesa (2017), the more experienced occupational therapist may not complete activity analyses on paper, as knowledge of the demands of activities becomes tacit and embedded into the occupational performance analysis process.

An activity analysis can help you identify the potential for change within an activity and the level of risk it might pose. It may be helpful to discuss your completed activity analysis with your educator, but it would not typically be something you would include in your client's occupational therapy documentation (as activity analysis provides a general understanding of how a task is performed and is not specific to an individual client).

ACTIVITY
....

Look at your priority occupation(s) from Chapter 7. Select one and complete an activity analysis using the template in Chapter 4 or one you are familiar with from your university learning. Discuss this with your peer and educator.

PLANNING FOR OUTCOME MEASUREMENT

It is important to think about how we might measure change *now*, as you cannot compare anything at the end of your occupational therapy involvement if you don't know how the client was doing his/her occupations when you started. In the OTIPM, outcome measurement is described as "Re-evaluate for enhanced and satisfying occupational performance" (see Chapter 13), and contains two key ways to measure if there has been a change after our intervention:

1   An observable change in occupational performance
2   A change in how satisfied the person (or significant others) is with his/her performance

ACTIVITY
....

Look at the information you have gathered so far when determining the occupational priorities. Consider what you know now and how you

might compare this at the end of your intervention. Could you measure changes in:
- The client's occupational performance?
- The client's satisfaction with occupational performance and/or level of participation in life roles?
- The environment where the occupation is performed?
- The occupational performance and/or satisfaction of significant others in the client constellation?

PREPARATIONS FOR OBSERVATIONS

BEING OCCUPATION-CENTRED

To work in an occupation-centred way, your assessment should focus on the person 'doing' his/her priority occupation(s). In developing the occupational profile and prioritising what is important to focus on, you will likely have gathered an array of information, including:

- The range of occupations a person does
- The patterns (routines) in which he/she performs the occupations
- The person's goals and aspirations
- The person's roles and responsibilities
- The environments in which the occupations are performed
- Who else is in the context
- The person's current and past health history

Being occupation-centred means that although we have all this information, we need to focus on how the person does his/her occupation(s) first. This means, where possible, doing an observation of the person doing the priority occupation. We will do this using an observation and occupational performance analysis, but there are other options available, such as those discussed for children in Chien and Brown (2017).

This may seem obvious, and it is clear within the OTIPM. We do, however, have many situations within occupational therapy practice where the focus shifts from the person doing the occupation, to a focus on assessing the person's underlying body functions/ structures or the environment and then making predictions about how these factors might impact on the person's occupational performance (see Chapter 2 for a discussion of top-down, bottom-up and top-to-bottom-up reasoning). While we are not stating that these factors are unimportant, we are saying that the *person doing the occupation* should be the first thing we do as occupational therapists, and only look at body functions/structure or environmental factors when they directly relate to the performance of an occupation. These factors will be addressed when we define the cause of the occupational performance challenges in Chapter 11.

There are many examples of assessments that assess underlying body functions/structures and you are likely to come across them during your placements. Remember that these tools measure levels of impairment and there is emerging evidence that the *degree of body function impairments are not good predictors of how someone will perform occupations*. This is because occupational performance arises out of a complex interaction between the person, the occupation and the environment. Knowing solely about impairment in the person is not sufficient.

ACTIVITY

Look at the assessment tools available in your setting. What is their primary focus?
- – Occupational performance?
- – Participation?
- – Impairment in body functions/structures?
- – Environment?

WHEN PEOPLE HAVE DIFFERENT PRIORITIES

We have said throughout this book that we must focus on the occupations which are important to the client. Sometimes, however, the person and the people supporting them will *prioritise different things and have different views about the person's level of difficulty*. In these cases, we need to negotiate between competing priority areas. For example, it might be that a child wishes to play football, while parents want her to organise her room and teachers want her to keep focused in class. You may decide to work on a priority area identified by each key person involved or you could negotiate with the group to focus on an initial target before moving on to the next occupation.

You will also have an opinion to share in these negotiations. As an occupational therapist, you may be able to anticipate the level of challenge or risk involved in an occupation (as you have completed an activity analysis and you understand about the person–environment–occupation interplay). You might, therefore, recommend starting with addressing safety concerns associated with an occupation, or with occupations that involve only small or straightforward changes to improve performance.

WHEN PEOPLE DO THINGS DIFFERENTLY IN DIFFERENT CONTEXTS

We know that the person's occupational performance is influenced by the interplay among person, environment and occupation. At times, you may *want to see the same occupation but in different contexts,* to help you understand the impact the environment has on the person's occupational performance. For example, a person may be able to get washed, dressed and use the toilet when they are in hospital, but they are unable to do this when he/she gets home. Another example might be where a person can talk with others in a regular church group, but struggles to have conversations with work colleagues. Observing in different contexts or situations can help you identify the environmental conditions which facilitate the person's occupational performance, which might then be trialled in different scenarios.

Sometimes, you may assess an occupation the person does well. This can help identify what supports an occupation to be successful, which could be applied to less successful occupations. Moreover, you may find some people are only agreeable initially to you observing something they know they can do well. This can be an effective way to build rapport and trust with the person, so that he/she later feels comfortable in you observing something that he/she finds difficult.

WHEN IT IS NOT APPROPRIATE TO OBSERVE

There are examples of where it *may not be appropriate for you to observe* the priority occupation. For example, you may be working with a person from a cultural or religious group where it would not be appropriate for you to observe them conducting personal care because of your gender. Although this is not ideal, you may decide to observe something else to give you a general idea about the client's performance and then use this information, along with reports from the person or relevant others, to make recommendations.

THINKING ABOUT RISK

Occupational therapists need to consider potential risks associated with assessments and interventions. As a student, you also need to be aware of and assess risks relating to how the person performs his/her occupations.

You may be required to complete specific risk assessments. Some of these will need to be completed before an observational assessment can take place. For example, in forensic mental health services you will need to do a formal risk assessment before engaging in a cooking assessment where sharp knives are used. For these types of risk assessments, there are often templates which need to be completed. Seek guidance from your educator as required.

As you are doing your assessment, you may also identify other risks. For example, there is out-of-date food in the fridge, the person's front door is not fully secure or the person isn't taking his/her prescribed medication. Depending on the person and his/her circumstances, you may have a duty to act on these risks. Discuss your obligations with your educator so that you can be guided as to the best thing to do.

When thinking about risk, consider this general risk assessment/management process:

1   Recognise the hazard and the potential risk.
2   Assess the likelihood, degree and nature of the risk.
    - How might the risk be triggered?
    - Who is at risk and how?
    - How severe is the risk?
    - How likely is it to happen?
    - Does the benefit of the client doing the occupation mean the risk is considered reasonable?
3   Develop, record and review a risk management plan.
    - How could risks or triggers be reduced, avoided or eliminated altogether?
    - What should happen if the risk became a reality and an incident occurred?
    - What are the potential consequences of the person not doing this occupation?

ACTIVITY
....

In planning your observation, answer the following questions (McILwain, 2006) about risk.
1   **Identify what could go wrong:**
    - *Analyse* how often this might occur.
    - *Try* to eliminate the risk.
2   **Identify what could happen:**
    - *Analyse* how severe the effect would be.
    - *Try* to avoid the risk.

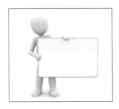

EDUCATOR EXAMPLES HERE:
RISK ASSESSMENT
....

-   Where available, provide examples of risk assessment templates and completed examples which are used in the setting.

IDENTIFYING WHERE TO OBSERVE

Where possible, assessment of occupation should happen where the person would usually perform this occupation. In practice, however, this is not always possible. If you are in a situation where you must assess someone in an environment which isn't where they would usually perform, you should be mindful that *the environment will impact on what you see.*

For example, observing a person performing in a hospital kitchen environment which is well organised, well stocked with fully functioning equipment, and distraction free, may not give you a good indication of how that person will perform in a home environment which is cluttered and disorganised, with limited equipment available and lots of distractions. Always consider the interplay among person, environment and occupation and be cautious in the reporting of your recommendations if you have not seen the person in his/her usual setting.

There will be times, however, where a different environment is the 'usual' setting for a person. For example, if a person is in hospital (particularly if they are there for a while), then this is his/her usual context for the time being. Enabling a person to make his/her own cup of tea in the hospital kitchen or play a game of cards in the lounge area in the hospital is important for his/her health and well-being *now*. When it is time to go home, you can then focus on how these occupations might be transferred.

IDENTIFYING WHEN TO OBSERVE

Where possible, try and see the person *do the occupation at the usual time* he/she would do it or at the time he/she has identified as being a problem. For example, try to observe personal care first thing in the morning or when he/she usually does this, or observe mealtimes at the person's usual time.

There will be instances, however, where this is not possible. For example, it is probably not practical to observe toileting in the middle of the night. In these situations, it is likely you will have to observe toileting during the day and make a best guess about how night time is different.

Some of the people we work with may be flexible and willing to be observed doing an occupation at another time in the day (e.g. they may be willing to get dressed and undressed in the middle of the day). In this situation, be mindful that changing the time of day can impact on the person's performance.

In other situations, it would be difficult to observe at an atypical time. For example, some people with a learning disability or who have autism may not perform well when asked to do something outside of their usual routines. In these instances, if you cannot be there at the time it is usually done, then you may ask someone else to observe who is there at the time they usually do it (e.g. a support worker or family member) and discuss the observations with them afterwards.

USING TECHNOLOGY

In some settings, short videos could be made or someone might be observed over an internet video system. For example, if it is not appropriate or possible for you to be in a person's home during an evening meal, you may be able to observe some aspects via video.

Be aware that using video can distract a person or make him/her feel anxious or uncomfortable. Also, you do not want to obsess with observing the video over and over, as you will see far more (and hence see many more problems) than you would in a 'real-life' situation.

Permissions would need to be sought to record observations from the people who will appear in the video and from any manager of settings in which they take place (e.g. the manager of a residential care home). You will also need to think about how you would store the data securely and for how long you will need to keep it.

THINKING ABOUT CONSENT

Each setting will have its own policy on how and when to gain consent from clients and, if appropriate, parents or carers. There is also likely to be a legal framework which you need to follow, such as the Mental Capacity Act (2005) in the United Kingdom.

In general, you should document:

- That consent was gained
- From whom it was gained (e.g. parent/guardian for a child or the person themselves for an adult)
- How this was done (e.g. verbally, signing a form)

If a person cannot consent, consider and clearly document how you believe your assessment and intervention will be in his/her best interest. There may also be mental capacity guidance that you need to adhere to. Be aware that it is unlikely that someone else can consent for another adult.

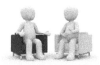

ACTIVITY

....

Consider the following questions about consent and use them as a basis for discussion in supervision:
- Do you know who you will be working with at this stage or is it still being negotiated?
- Will you be working with the whole setting/one aspect (such as a class)/ small group/or individual clients? Will this make a difference to the consent you will need?
- Will expectations be raised about what you might be able to provide? What might happen if you are unable to meet those expectations?
- Who do you need to gain consent from? How will you gain consent?

CARRYING OUT OBSERVATIONS

What makes occupational therapy unique from other professionals is how we observe and analyse occupational performance. The client's perception of his/her occupational performance is important (and this is gathered on the occupational performance analysis form), but it is often not sufficient to base interventions upon this alone. Research has highlighted that there is often a discrepancy between a client's view of his/her occupational strengths and needs and what observational assessment identifies (Nielsen and Wæhrens, 2015; Wæhrens, Bliddal, Danneskiold-Samsøe, Lund and Fisher, 2012). Therefore, both client and observational perceptions are equally important. In this section, we will explore practical considerations when undertaking observational assessments.

As guided by the OTIPM, this next section will focus on using an occupational performance analysis (as introduced in Chapter 4) to gather and interpret our observations. To help us consider occupational performance in sufficient detail, we use the skill item descriptors introduced in Chapter 4. You could use other observational tools at this stage in the OTIPM and you may wish to discuss the options with your educator. We will continue to use the occupational performance analysis in this and subsequent chapters, as we wish to maintain a logical flow to support your understanding of the occupational therapy process.

TAKING NOTES WHILE OBSERVING

It will not be possible to complete an occupational performance analysis form during an observation as it will be necessary to refer to guidance on the relevant performance skills. While observing, it is therefore usual to write down in brief notes what the client was doing and the order in which it happened. This helps to capture the temporal organisation of the performance (How long did each step take? Did they repeat a step? Was the sequence logical? etc.). These notes will then be used to complete the occupational performance analysis and later the occupational therapy report (see Chapter 9). An example of notes (adapted from Fisher, Bryze, Hume and Griswold, 2007) follows:

> Reached for tray
> Reached for cutlery – put on tray
> Looked away – pause – cutlery fell off tray
> Picked up cutlery – fumbled
> Walked to counter
> Long pause – teacher asked which meal? – wait long pause
> Child no answer – looked away
> Given plate of food
> Child put plate on tray – tray wobbled – plate almost fell
> Cutlery fell off tray – teacher picked it up
> Child walked with tray to table – teacher followed closely
> Long pause – looked around – high noise level in the room
> Sat down then put tray on table

Picked up knife and fork
Stabbed sausage with knife
Sausage slipped from plate

You should discuss your intention to write notes with the client beforehand. If he/she is concerned about this, being able to read what you have written at the end can be reassuring. It is not recommended that memory is relied upon, as it's likely details will be forgotten and it is practically not always possible to have time immediately after assessment to document everything in sufficient detail. However, there may be instances where it is not appropriate to write notes, such as in a hospital situation with infection control concerns or where it creates a large amount of anxiety for the client. In these circumstances, it may help to have time immediately after the assessment to make good notes.

Your observation notes may not need to be included in the client's file, but are working notes to support the completion of an occupational performance analysis template. Check your local policies, but the occupational performance analysis template and report will be stored in the client's file. You will need to consider, however, where you store your initial rough notes, what identifiable information is on them and how/when you will dispose of these.

GIVING INITIAL FEEDBACK

As we discussed in Chapter 6 it is important to give some feedback to the person after the observation to aid in your rapport building. Formal feedback of assessment is often done after you have analysed your data. There are times, however, where you will have some initial recommendations which you could discuss immediately.

For example, you might note when doing an assessment in a residential facility that the TV and radio are on in the sitting room and this is distracting for many residents; you may therefore suggest turning one source of sound off. Another example might be you observe a staff member move someone in a way that isn't as safe as it could be. In this case, you would want to discuss safer ways for moving the client as soon as possible. The purpose of these initial suggestions is to demonstrate what you have been working on and, if appropriate, the management of any safety issues.

USING THE OCCUPATIONAL PERFORMANCE ANALYSIS IN A GROUP

The OTIPM provides an occupational therapy process which is designed for working with individual clients. It can, however, also work well if you are focusing on the needs of more than one person. This could happen on role-established, role-emerging or project placements. Gathering information and prioritising occupational needs would be based on discussions with group members. For example, it may be identified that the mealtimes in a residential facility or the playground in a school are the main concerns for the group.

Observing in a group situation can be challenging as we need the level of detail provided by an occupational performance analysis to reason our interventions, but this tool is designed for observing an individual. To overcome this issue, it may be helpful to focus on one client for 15–20 minutes, then observe the activity again, this time focusing on a different client. Staff members or clients in the setting can indicate which people would be most suitable to observe to give an overall indication of the issues experienced. Comparing the occupational performance analyses for the individual clients can provide useful indicators of the successes and challenges experienced and enable you to reason your intervention recommendations. Further information on group observations can be found in Dancza, Missiuna and Pollock (2017).

There will be times when you are focusing on a person's ability to fulfil the social interaction demands of an occupation (e.g. buying lunch from a canteen, having a meeting with work colleagues, participating in a life skills group). In these situations, you will be observing at least two people simultaneously, i.e. your client and the person or people with whom he/she is interacting. It might be helpful to focus on your client, but also record what the social partner is doing. This will help in your interpretation of the cause of any challenges and the development of intervention strategies.

ADVICE FOR EDUCATORS IN SUPPORTING STUDENTS WITH DETAILED ASSESSMENTS

Your role in supporting students to undertake assessments will depend on the type of placement (role-established, role-emerging or project) and the placement setting. This section offers suggestions for you as an educator in supporting students undertake their assessments.

JOINT OR INDEPENDENT OBSERVATIONS

Observing together with students or letting them observe by themselves are both useful learning opportunities. In a role-emerging or project placement, you are unlikely to be present when students carry out their observations. Therefore, you are relying on the student's feedback of what he/she saw. This can be positive and negative. When students are required to explain in detail what they observed, they often clarify for themselves the essential elements and can identify parts which they missed. You are, however, less able to guide them during their observation and students cannot check the accuracy of their observations against a more experienced occupational therapist.

In a role-established setting where you may be present, you can compare your observations with the student, prompt the student to look for certain things or fill in the gaps if he/she missed something. Students, however, may rely on your guidance and may not practice articulating what they saw. Where possible try to have a mix of doing joint and independent observations.

ENCOURAGE PEER WORKING

If you are supporting two or more students on placement, they may benefit from opportunities to do joint and individual observations. When doing joint observations, students can compare what they saw. If doing individual observations, students can discuss with their peers what they observed to help them clarify their understanding of the performance. Having these discussions prior to supervision can help students shape their thoughts before they chat them through with you.

HELPING STUDENTS MAKE SENSE OF THEIR OCCUPATIONAL PERFORMANCE ANALYSIS

The process of translating rough notes onto the occupational performance analysis form helps students clarify what they observed and begin to interpret this information. This is, however, a notoriously challenging task for students as they are not sure what is important and what is not. Also, as they are becoming familiar with the skill items on the occupational performance analysis, they may report their observations in unexpected places or put too much or not enough emphasis on one aspect.

Talking through findings can be helpful for students. It is suggested that during these discussions you have the motor, process and social interaction skills item descriptions available (see Appendix 4.1). Ask about each skill item individually, for example:

- Did the child complete the essential task of writing a story? (Heeds)
- Did the child write the story with a logical sequence, such as pick up the pen, taking off the lid and then writing in one direction? (Sequences)
- Did the child pause before writing a word? (Initiates)
- Did the child pause in the middle of writing a word? (Continues)

When asking questions, use the text in the guidance notes and try to substitute the actual activity elements as shown here. As you are questioning the students, try to pull out the important aspects of the assessment and use your reasoning to emphasise the critical aspects to students.

USING OTHER ASSESSMENT TOOLS

Students have access to a range of assessment tools during placement and often find it challenging to reason when to use a tool or why they would choose one tool over another. We have presented some tools and where these would fit within the OTIPM (occupational profiling, activity analysis, occupational performance analysis, general observations sheet). You may guide students to use these and ask that they provide feedback to you about them. Students may also have been introduced to different tools at university or seen tools you use in your setting. It is important that students reason why they are using these tools, when to use them and what they will do with the results, before they use them with clients.

For example, after completing the occupational performance analysis, you may want to know about a person's body function/structure impairment as this can be helpful to understand the challenges experienced by the person. It is important to support students to use additional assessments when there is a rationale for doing so, i.e. questions remain following the observation about the potential causes of the performance issues (see Chapter 11 for further discussion).

Additional assessments might include assessments of motivation, mood, memory, sensory processing, balance, grip strength, range of movement, environment etc. These may be within the remit of occupational therapy, or it may be appropriate to refer to someone else whose remit these assessments are more aligned to (e.g. a psychologist carrying out a cognitive assessment, a psychiatric nurse or psychiatrist carrying out an assessment of mood or anxiety). Following the OTIPM steps, these additional assessments can happen where relevant in the "Clarify or interpret the reason(s) for client's problems of occupational performance" step (see Chapter 11)

There are also examples of environmental assessments that are conducted without the person being there (e.g. an access visit to a person's home prior to them being discharged from hospital). These may highlight general environmental hazards such as rugs being in situ, but it is important to reinforce to students that they will not give specific information about how a person will manage his/her occupations in this environment, nor how well he/she would navigate the environmental risks. Ideally you would assess the client in that environment. Where this is not possible, the student will need to be careful when making recommendations about ways to improve occupational performance as these will be based on estimates of the person's capacity to do the occupation in that environment.

In any of these situations, it is helpful if you are using the OTIPM to show students where these other assessment tools fit and discuss their focus (e.g. occupational performance, environment, body functions/structures etc.).

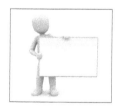

EDUCATOR EXAMPLES HERE:
ASSESSMENT TOOLS

– Provide examples for students of relevant observational tools or assessment materials which form part of your placement setting. Ask students to reflect also on their university learning for examples. Where possible, show students examples of completed assessment forms and templates so they can understand the expectations.

LEARNING THROUGH DOCUMENTATION

As students are carrying out assessment tasks, you may need to remind them to document what they are doing. Chapter 9 outlines how you might set up progress notes and report documentation as they relate to the OTIPM. You may have your established procedures which need to be followed. As with assessment tools, students are likely to benefit from examples to follow. Students also learn and consolidate their understanding of the occupational therapy process through summarising findings in a report. It is a good opportunity to start this now with a summary of the background information and assessment strategy.

CHAPTER SUMMARY

This chapter explored how the priority occupation(s) of a client can be analysed in detail using observation as the key assessment tool. We drew from Chapter 4 and the occupational profile, activity analysis and occupational performance analysis and considered how they could be used in a placement context. This included how to prepare for observations and carrying out observations. The chapter concluded with advice for educators to support students undertaking assessments.

REFERENCES

Chard G, Mesa S (2017) 'Analysis of occupational performance: Motor, process and social interaction skills'. In: M Curtin, J Adams, M Egan, eds, *Occupational therapy for people experiencing illness, injury or impairment: Promoting occupation and participation.* 7th edn. Edinburgh: Elsevier, pp. 217–243.

Chien CW, Brown T (2017) 'Assessing children's occupations and participation'. In: S Rodger, A Kennedy-Behr, eds, *Occupation-centred practice with children: A practical guide for occupational therapists.* 2nd edn. West Sussex, UK: Wiley-Blackwell, pp. 133–163.

Dancza KM, Missiuna C, Pollock N (2017) 'Occupation-centred practice: When the classroom or the school is your client'. In: S Rodger, A Kennedy-Behr, eds, *Occupation-centred practice with children: A practical guide for occupational therapists.* 2nd edn. West Sussex, UK: Wiley-Blackwell, pp. 257–287.

Department of Health (2005) *Mental capacity act.* London, UK: Crown Copyright.

Fisher AG (2009) *Occupational Therapy intervention process model: A model for planning and implementing top-down, client centred, and occupation-based interventions.* Fort Collins, CO: Three Star Press.

Fisher AG, Bryze K, Hume V, Griswold L (2007) *School AMPS: School version of the assessment of motor and process skills.* 2nd edn. Fort Collins, CO: Three Star Press, Inc.

McILwain JC (2006) 'A review: A decade of clinical risk management and risk tools'. *Clinician in Management, 14*(4), 189–199.

Nielsen K, Wæhrens EE (2015) 'Occupational therapy evaluation: Use of self report and/or observation?'. *Scandinavian Journal of Occupational Therapy, 22*(1), 13–23.

Wæhrens EE, Bliddal H, Danneskiold-Samsøe B, Lund H, Fisher AG (2012) 'Differences between questionnaire- and interview-based measures of activities of daily living (ADL) ability and their association with observed ADL ability in women with rheumatoid arthritis, knee osteoarthritis, and fibromyalgia'. *Scandinavian Journal of Rheumatology, 41,* 95–102.

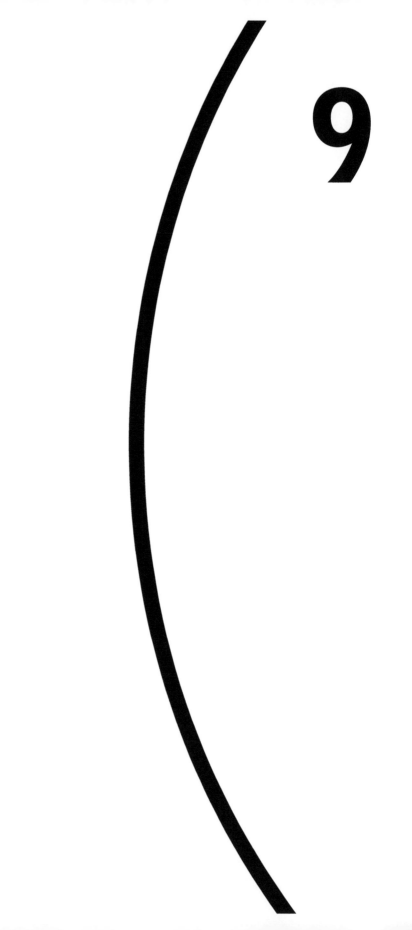

CHAPTER 9
DEFINING AND DESCRIBING TASK ACTIONS THE CLIENT DOES AND DOES NOT PERFORM EFFECTIVELY (DOCUMENTATION)

Karina Dancza and Jodie Copley

INTENDED CHAPTER OUTCOMES

By the end of this chapter, readers will have an overview of:

- The purpose of documentation and how it can support reasoning
- How to ensure that documentation is occupation-centred and client-friendly
- Key considerations to tailor your notes and reports for different contexts
- Two documentation styles: progress notes and reports

STAGE IN THE OTIPM

As an occupational therapist, it is important that work is informed by practice models such as the Occupational Therapy Intervention Process Model (OTIPM; Fisher, 2009). In this chapter, we are discussing how to make sense of your assessment and document your practice (Figure 9.1). Please take a few moments to revisit the OTIPM diagram now to familiarise yourself with the concepts in this phase of the OTIPM framework.

INTRODUCTION

You have spent considerable time becoming familiar with your placement setting and potential clients. Your observational assessment provided detail about the priority occupational areas. Now it is time to consolidate and document this information. In the OTIPM, this stage is indicated by the box labelled "Define and describe task actions the client does and does not perform effectively."

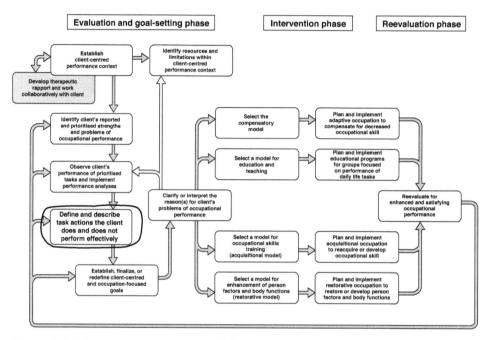

Figure 9.1 Schematic representation of the steps in the OTIPM: Define and describe task actions the client does and does not perform effectively

Adapted from Fisher (2009). Available: www.innovativeotsolutions.com/content/wp-content/uploads/2014/01/English-OTIPM-handout.pdf. Reprinted with permission.

While documentation is indicated in only one box on the OTIPM, you will need to record your observations, plans and actions throughout the occupational therapy process. Even though you haven't yet finished the occupational therapy process, it is recommended that you start your report(s) now so that you keep up with what you are doing and not wait until later in your placement to begin writing.

PURPOSE OF DOCUMENTATION

Documentation is a requirement of being a professional (Royal College of Occupational Therapists [RCOT], 2015; Simpson, 1998). Documentation has a range of purposes, including:

- Providing a means of communicating amongst team members in an organisation, between organisations and between professionals and clients
- Recording your reasoning, which allows you to justify your therapy decisions
- Meeting the policy and procedure requirements of the organisation (including evidencing the service for funding arrangements)

More than that, it is a valuable way to clarify your thinking and assist your decision making. Report writing is like any skill you learn: the more practice you have and the more constructive feedback you receive, the better you will become at it.

Documentation requirements vary between practice settings. You will need to investigate the legal requirements and your service setting's policies relating to the production, storage and disposal of your notes, reports and any other information you hold (including information in your electronic diary, mobile phone, photographs/video recordings, etc.).

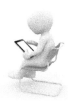

ACTIVITY

Make a note of the questions you have about documentation. Speak with your educator and university placement coordinator to ensure that you are compliant with local rules about documentation.

FORMAT AND CONTENT FOR OCCUPATION-CENTRED DOCUMENTATION

Our professional values and role within a team are highlighted in our documentation. The format, length and level of detail required in your documentation is influenced by its purpose and intended audience. You may need to follow an established structure and headings for your documentation. For example, in some hospital settings, the SOAP format is used (Subjective, Objective, Assessment, Plan), while in community settings the notes may be structured around client goals.

Donaldson, McDermott, Hollands, Copley and Davidson (2004) interviewed parents about what they wanted in occupational therapy and speech pathology reports for their children. They found that parents were not concerned with report length, provided the information was clear. As one parent commented: 'I don't care if it was ten pages long as long as it was explained. . . . I'd rather read two more pages and understand it than read two less pages and not have a clue" (p. 32).

Any time we write, it is useful to keep in mind two golden rules:

1 The client can read and understand what we have written.
2 We write about occupation, explaining the reasons why particular issues with occupational performance are occurring and how these might be addressed.

WRITING PROGRESS NOTES

Writing progress notes is a way of tracking your reasoning and actions for yourself and others. It is an essential part of your work throughout the occupational therapy process (not just at this stage in the OTIPM).

You will need to either follow the setting's usual practices (e.g. documenting in medical charts, therapy files or electronic records), or in a role-emerging setting create your own way of recording your involvement. You may also need to consider if you are going to add to an existing set of notes or create independent notes. If there are other students from different disciplines on placement at the same time as you, consider if you will have separate or joint notes.

Progress notes can take many forms and it is important that you discuss the specific requirements of the setting with your educator. For example, you may keep notes for individual clients or groups of clients, depending on your priority areas. In either instance, you can divide notes into two parts:

1   Notes describing information gathered, written in chronological order, such as discussions with staff members and clients and observations of priority occupations
2   Additional documents (such as assessment forms or occupational performance analysis notes)

PROGRESS NOTES FOR INDIVIDUAL CLIENTS

It is perhaps most common for progress notes to be created for individual clients. There are standards for notes which need to be maintained. For paper notes it is common to have each page clearly identifiable, pages numbered, dated and signed for each entry, etc. Electronic records will often dictate the information required. Refer to your university notes, consider your previous placements and consult with any relevant documents about record keeping (such as The Royal College of Occupational Therapists in the United Kingdom, www.rcot.co.uk). If you have not seen relevant examples for your setting, refer to Table 9.1 to review a sample structure for notes for an individual child in a school setting.

PROGRESS NOTES FOR AN OCCUPATIONAL CONTEXT

In some circumstances, it may be appropriate to generate group notes about a specific occupational context, such as a school playground, aged-care residence recreation room or hospital canteen. This might be particularly relevant if you are working to make universal changes to a setting for the benefit of all clients.

To document this type of work, you could create an occupational therapy notes folder with a section for each priority area (see Table 9.2). Be aware that in some circumstances you may not be able to use names of individual clients as it could be a breach of confidentiality. Regardless, you still need to ensure the storage of these notes is safe as they may contain sensitive information.

Table 9.1 Documentation format for an individual

Name: Nicole Taylor **Date of birth:** 08/04/11 **Classroom**: year 1 – Badger's class
Page: 1 of 1 **Class teacher**: Mrs Hancock **Classroom assistants**: Mrs O'Reilly

Date	Activity	Name/Signature
14/4/17	Observations of children getting changed for PE – school context observation form completed (see classroom notes for details). During this observation, it was noted that Nicole was considerably slower than her peers in changing for PE and she required frequent teacher assistance. **Plan:** To discuss observations with Mrs Hancock.	Flynn Dare (third year occupational therapy student)
15/4/17	Discussion with Mrs Hancock. She reported concerns with Nicole's fine motor skills which she thought were impacting on her ability to get dressed. She also reported that Nicole was often distracted and was constantly losing her belongings. Mrs Hancock wants Nicole to keep up with the class when changing for PE and agreed it was suitable for the occupational therapy students to progress with a detailed observation following parental consent. **Plan:** Permission form sent to parents via a letter.	Flynn Dare (third year occupational therapy student)
19/4/11	Permission received from parents (see file). Spoke with Nicole. Explained the role of the occupational therapist and asked her how she finds doing school tasks. She highlighted that she wanted to be quicker changing for PE and that she wanted to learn to skip with a skipping rope. She reported that she found drawing and art fun and she felt she was really good at this. Spoke with Mrs Hancock and arranged a time to observe changing for PE on 22/4/17. Arranged to observe Nicole in the playground when the skipping ropes were available. **Plan:** Complete two observations	Flynn Dare (third year occupational therapy student)
22/4/17	A detailed observation was completed for Nicole (see occupational analysis form for details). Key observations noted: – There was very little space for Nicole to change and she was not able to sit down to dress. – Nicole looked away frequently to the other children in the room. – Nicole needed teacher assistance to search and locate her belongings, which were in another child's space. – Nicole put on her jumper before putting on her shirt (i.e. sequences). **Plan:** To discuss observations with long-arm supervisor and consider the potential causes of the difficulties. These will be formulated into an interim report. Meet with Mrs Hancock to discuss the findings and to set a goal.	Flynn Dare (third year occupational therapy student)

Table 9.2 Documentation format for a group

General/classroom notes: year 1   **Class teacher:** Mrs Worthington   **Page:** 1 of 1
Classroom assistants: Mrs Temme (Mon–Wed) and Ms Newbury (Thur, Fri)

Date	Activity	Name/Signature
10/4/17	School context observation completed for year 1 classroom (see additional notes). Spoke with Mrs Worthington about her classroom. She identified the following priority areas for the children in her class: – Getting changed for PE – Keeping focused during carpet time **Plan:** Observe the children changing for PE on 14/4/17 and carpet time on 18/4/17.	Holly Johnson (third year occupational therapy student)
14/4/17	Observations of children getting changed for PE. School context observation sheet completed (see attached form). Key observations noted: – The noise level was intense. – Lots of belongings around the classroom. – No clear spaces for children's belongings. – One child was very slow changing for PE and needed constant prompts. **Plan:** To complete an additional observation and occupational performance analysis of one child who was noted to be much slower than the others (see individual children's file for further details). To discuss with the teacher the observations and consider workable solutions.	Holly Johnson (third year occupational therapy student) Flynn Dare (third year occupational therapy student)
18/4/17	Observations completed of carpet time. Key findings included the length of time children spend on the carpet, the space available and seating options for children. See attached observational notes for additional detail. **Plan:** Discuss observations with class teacher-planned for 19/4/17.	Flynn Dare (third year occupational therapy student)

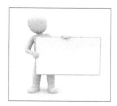

EDUCATOR EXAMPLES HERE:
PROGRESS NOTES

– Where possible, provide students with examples of progress notes and templates on which you would like them to base their own notes.

TO COUNTER-SIGN OR NOT TO COUNTER-SIGN . . .

In some circumstances, it may be a requirement for your notes to be counter-signed (or co-signed) by your educator or other qualified occupational therapist. Check within your setting as to the exact process and format for this (such as counter-signing each entry or each page of notes). Some placement settings have found it helpful to clearly identify notes as associated with student learning activities, particularly if the supervisor has not witnessed the action taking place (as would be typical on role-emerging placements). In these situations, the following statement could be included in the notes:

> "These notes reflect the supervision discussions which occurred between the occupational therapy students and the occupational therapy supervisor."

In other situations, the student may have been delegated the activity of writing the note and is therefore deemed competent to do so without a counter-signature (RCOT, 2015). In all cases, however, it is important that you identify yourself as an occupational therapy student (and not an occupational therapist), at least until you graduate!

WRITING REPORTS

At times during your work you will need to account for your reasoning and actions in a more formal way, such as in a report. There are many report formats you can use. Your intended audience will help determine the preferred format, although it is important to remember that if your writing is client/family-friendly, it will also likely be professional-friendly.

Research on report writing often comes from psychology, although there is some literature within occupational therapy (e.g. Donaldson et al., 2004; Groth-Marnat and Horvath, 2006; Harvey, 2006; Makepeace and Zwicker, 2014; Mastoras, Climie, McCrimmon and Schwean, 2011). Common issues include:

- Poor readability
- Generic interpretations
- Test-by-test reporting and reliance on test scores
- Poor links between referral questions and results/recommendations
- Focus on client weaknesses

Ways to avoid the common report-writing traps include:

1 Address the client's/caregiver's main concerns/priorities and write in an occupation-centred way (see the 'two golden rules' previously described).
2 Make it reader friendly.
   - Avoid jargon.
   - Use an appropriate level of explanation.
   - Use clear and simple wording.

3   Address strengths as well as weaknesses.
    –   Provide a balanced and comprehensive picture of the client.
4   Give a clear follow-up plan.
    –   Suggest specific, practical strategies (with some flexibility as you may not know exactly what will work until you try it!).

The following sections provide a step-by-step guide to creating a report, following the OTIPM framework. While initially developed for students on role-emerging placements, this guide may also be helpful to those on role-established placements if the organisation is open to this report writing style. Every situation is different and you need to alter your report format to meet the needs of the client and setting. Therefore, the headings here may need to be adapted.

As an example, throughout this section we will refer to John, who is a child in a school classroom. You may also wish to refer to Appendix 9.1, which is a completed report for Lee (the case study used in Chapter 4 to illustrate the occupational performance analysis).

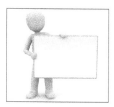

EDUCATOR EXAMPLES HERE: REPORTS

–   Where possible, provide students with examples of reports on which you would like them to base their own reports.

INTRODUCTION TO THE REPORT

Identify the document as an occupational therapy report (or interdisciplinary report if that is the case). Clearly state when the report was written and who the report is about. Common demographic headings include:

–   Date of report
–   Name of client
–   Date of birth
–   Age

You might want to add other identifying information such as a client number, classroom/ward name and parent/carer details (particularly if it is a child or vulnerable adult). Check with your educator and relevant people within the placement context about how to identify your report.

Another important consideration is how you *label each page of your report*. Think about what is needed if the report was printed and pages separated. Name of client, date of birth, client number, date and page number could be useful in a header/footer.

State why you became involved. This could be from an initial referral or a concern raised. Try to keep this factual, concise and focused on the occupational needs. For example:

"**Initial concern:** Mrs Hill, school Special Educational Needs Coordinator, expressed concerns with John's handwriting and paying attention in class. This concern was discussed with John's parents and a referral was made to occupational therapy via John's General Practitioner. The reason for occupational therapy involvement was to find out ways to help John keep focused in class, particularly when he needs to write."

Provide relevant background context, such as pertinent health or developmental history, people in the client's life, diagnosis, etc. You will need to be selective in what you report, as you do not need to re-state everything that is written elsewhere (e.g. in other reports/ letters). Always remember that the client and family will read this report. When making decisions about what to include in background information, ask yourself:

– What is my occupational therapy focus? (i.e. what occupations am I considering?)
– What is relevant in the person's history which *relates closely* to these priority occupations?
– What information is sensitive, but should be reported (e.g. diagnosis, challenging family situation)?
– What information is sensitive, but is not relevant to the occupations I am considering (e.g. history of counselling, sexual orientation) and therefore not to be included?
– Am I confident in the source of this background information and have I stated who has reported it? Be careful that it is not an unconfirmed diagnosis suggested in another report or incorrect information about a family situation,
– What is confidential and should not be repeated in my report?

For example, in John's report the background information that was stated included:

"**Background information:** Following interviews with John, his parents and teachers, it was reported that John enjoys school, although he does find completing his work challenging at times, particularly when it involves handwriting. John reported that he wants to be a Vet in the future as he loves animals. John's parents report that he has never enjoyed drawing, colouring or writing at home. Parents reported John received a diagnosis of Attention Deficit Hyperactivity Disorder and Developmental Coordination Disorder in April 2017. His vision and hearing have been checked (January 2017) with no reported concerns.

John's teacher described him as an able reader who enjoys science and maths. He has friends at school but does not always join in with the children playing football at lunchtime."

Finally, state the occupational therapy focus of the report. This will relate to the priority occupational area(s) you have identified and will be reflected in your occupational performance analysis. If there has been more than one area of focus, these will become your headings within the report e.g. making friends, gardening, housework. For example, in John's report it was written as:

"**Focus for occupational therapy assessment:** John completing his English work, consisting of writing an advertisement in the lesson prior to lunch."

ACTIVITY
....

Use an existing structure, or create a report template for yourself including the relevant title, headings and header/footer. Add the information you have gathered so far about the client(s) you are seeing. Use this as a discussion point in your supervision.

MAKING SENSE OF YOUR OCCUPATIONAL PERFORMANCE ANALYSIS

Once you have this introductory information in your report, the next stage is to add in the information you have gathered through your assessment. Fisher (2009) describes this in the OTIPM as "Define and describe task actions the client does and does not perform effectively". In practice, this means that once you have completed your detailed observations (see Chapter 8) you need to make sense of what you saw.

Completing the activity analysis and occupational performance analysis ensures that you have an in-depth understanding of how the occupation was performed and the potential for change to improve this performance. Your occupational performance analysis notes, in their raw form, are not written in a way which is meaningful to others. Therefore, these notes need to be analysed, filtered and reported in a way that can be universally understood. The next sections will describe how you can report on each aspect of the occupational performance analysis.

OVERALL QUALITY OF PERFORMANCE

The occupational performance analysis directs you to consider how the person performed overall during the observations of their occupational tasks. This is indicated by how you rated the person's overall quality of performance in terms of effort (motor), efficiency (process), social interaction, safety and need for assistance (Fisher, 2009 and see Chapter 4). When writing this baseline, remember to use the words which describe the rating you gave so that you can compare this at the re-evaluation stage. For example:

"John showed a *mild degree* of physical difficulty, a *moderate degree* of undesirable use of time and *frequent* need for verbal and physical prompts to complete the writing task. There was *no evidence* of risk for personal injury or environmental damage. There was some *minimal delay* in writing his advertisement due to his social skills."

ACTIVITY

....

Write your baseline statement and add it into your report.

SATISFACTION WITH OCCUPATIONAL PERFORMANCE

The occupational performance analysis has space to record how the client and relevant others felt about the occupational performance. Understanding the person's perspective of how they performed can provide useful information when thinking about priorities, goals and planning effective interventions. Try to remain focused on *the specific occupation* you have observed. For example:

"**John's satisfaction with his school work:** John reported that doing his work like his classmates was important to him. He said he was pleased with his writing but was looking forward to typing it on the computer.

John's teacher's satisfaction with his school work: John is required to complete his English work to meet the requirements of the national curriculum relating to developing imaginative skills. She suspects that John could have written more during the time allocated in class, although she was happy with his ideas."

ACTIVITY

....

Summarise the client and relevant others' satisfaction with performance in your report template.

ENVIRONMENT AND TASK OBJECTS

The people reading your report may not have been present during the assessment. Therefore, you need to describe aspects of the environment and task objects that are relevant to the person's occupational performance. Focus on what was relevant, rather than describing every detail. In John's example, the distractions in the environment were significant in how he attended during the lesson, so the summary focused on this aspect:

"Classroom environment and task objects

John's classroom has a variety of brightly coloured displays including a papermache 'spider' hanging from the ceiling. John sat at a group desk with four other children and there was no clear distinction between children's work areas.

John's position at the group desk was near the drawers. At times, it was difficult for the children to move past John's chair to access the drawers without knocking into him."

ACTIVITY
....

Summarise the relevant environment and task objects in your report template.

CREATING CLUSTERS

Your report so far has featured summaries of information about the person (history, perspectives) and the environment. The next step is to understand and interpret your observations of the *occupational performance*. The occupational performance analysis has directed you to consider the motor, process and social interaction skill items. This is to help you see the detail and consider the complexity of occupational performance.

Now you need to determine which skill item combinations were positively or negatively impacting on the person's performance. The following steps can help you think through this:

1   On your completed occupational performance analysis, highlight relative strengths of the motor, process and social interaction skill items (indicated by the boxes in the example on Table 9.3) and around 10–15 skill items which most significantly impacted on the person's occupational performance (indicated by the asterisk in the example in Table 9.3).
2   Group the skill items together to form clusters based on what you saw during the observation. Think of which step was happening when the skill item was observed to be a strength or problem. For example, talking about Star Wars was a problem for John and this was illustrated in the Questions and Transitions skill items. Questions and Transitions would be considered a 'cluster'.

Table 9.3 Example of highlighting strengths and areas of challenge in an occupational performance analysis (social interaction skills section)

Social Interaction Skills		
Skill item Please indicate in the adjacent box (*) if a skill item caused significant challenge to the occupational performance.		**Description of key observations**
Initiating and terminating social interaction – Approaches/starts – Concludes/disengages		John initiated a conversation with his peer which mildly disrupted the other child, but how he started and ended the conversation was effective.
Produces social interaction – Produces speech – Gesticulates – Speaks fluently		John spoke appropriately to his teacher and classmate. Use of gestures was appropriate. John spoke fluently with an appropriate pace.
Physically supporting social interaction – Turns toward – Looks – Places self – Touches – Regulates		John turned his body towards his classmate when talking with him. He did not turn toward his teacher when she was talking, but she was talking over his shoulder and both were focused on his work. John looked to his peer when talking to him. John placed himself very close to his peer when talking with him. The peer moved back slightly. No concerns were noted about responding to or initiated touch and no unusual impulses.
Shaping content of social interaction – Questions – Replies – Discloses – Expresses emotions – Disagrees – Thanks	*	John asked irrelevant questions to his peer about his favourite Star Wars characters. John replies and shares information with his teacher and peer appropriately. No concerns were noted with how John expressed his emotions or differences of opinion. John thanked the support teacher for the tissue.

(Continued)

Table 9.3 (Continued)

Maintaining flow of social interaction – Transitions – Time response – Times duration – Takes turns	*	John persisted in talking about Star Wars when it was not appropriate. John replied to conversation without hesitation. John spoke for a reasonable time to his peer and realised when he should get back to his own work. John took turns when talking with his peer and with the teacher.
Verbally supporting social interaction – Matches language – Clarifies – Acknowledges/encourages – Empathizes		John's language was appropriate for his teacher and peer. No issues were noted with John's understanding of his peer's comprehension. John acknowledged and encouraged his peer. No concerns were noted with John's ability to empathize.
Adapting social interaction – Heeds – Accommodates – Benefits		John could carry out and complete the intended purposes of his social interaction. John did not modify his social interaction when he saw that his peer was not interested in talking about Star Wars. John continued asking about Star Wars so he did not benefit from his peer ignoring him.

3. For each cluster, write a description of what you saw happen. Try to use regular language and not the jargon associated with the occupational performance analysis as this is not meaningful to most people. For the two clusters identified for John, you could write:

"Replies, takes turns, thanks

John replied to questions from both his teacher and peer and took turns when asking and answering questions. He also thanked the Learning Support Assistant for getting him a tissue.

Questions, transitions

John asked his classmates irrelevant questions about Star Wars. However, this only disrupted his performance for a brief time."

Some examples of clusters which could be created from John's process skill items (not listed in Table 9.3) could include:

Attends

John frequently looked away from what he was doing and he needed prompts to complete his work.

Initiates, continues

John paused frequently before writing the next word and while writing his words which also interfered with his task performance.

ACTIVITY
....

Create clusters from what you thought was relevant during your observation. There are no set number of clusters you should create, but Lee's report in Appendix 9.1 will give you some indication.

COMPLETING THE REPORT

At this stage in the occupational therapy process and the OTIPM, you will not be able to finalise the report with the information you currently have. You will need to keep adding to your report as you progress, so you may like to come back to this section later.

ESTABLISH, FINALIZE OR REDEFINE CLIENT-CENTRED AND OCCUPATION-FOCUSED GOALS

After you have a comprehensive picture of the client's occupational performance by creating your clusters, the next step in the OTIPM is to consolidate the goals with the person and relevant others. Setting goals and targets of therapy will focus your involvement and can be used as a comparison measure at the end (see Chapter 10 for guidance on goal setting). An example for John could be:

"Goal (in John's words): To keep up with my friends in class.

Target (reframed by the occupational therapist, John and his teacher): For John to be able to write his English story within the time allocated during the lesson, by the end of term (seven weeks)."

CLARIFY OR INTERPRET THE REASON(S) FOR CLIENT'S PROBLEMS OF OCCUPATIONAL PERFORMANCE

It is not enough to describe what happened during your observation. You also need to think about *why it happened*. Chapter 11 offers a variety of ways to help you to think about the potential causes of the occupational performance challenges you observed.

Once you have done this, write under each cluster *why* you think it happened. Look at the detail from the activity analysis to consider which parts of the task might be contributing. Also, include the information you have gathered from the background information, diagnosis, the social and physical environment or the client's perceptions/motivation for the task (see the arrows on the OTIPM). In John's example, it could be:

"Questions, transitions interpretation

John may be particularly interested in Star Wars and prefer to engage in this topic, rather than the school work task.

Attends interpretation

When John was looking away he appeared to be looking at the other children and displays around the room. It may be that his position in the classroom means that he can see all that is happening which distracts him from his work.

Initiates, continues interpretation

John paused when writing words to get a working pen to use. John said that he wanted to use words that he didn't know how to spell and this slowed him down. John was also interrupted with the frequent instructions given throughout the task."

INTERVENTION PHASE

The potential causes of the performance challenges will guide you to consider suitable intervention approaches. By sharing these ideas with the person, family and significant others, you can collaboratively devise intervention options which will support occupational performance. Chapter 12 outlines considerations when planning and carrying out interventions. Documentation of strategies should be clearly related to your interpretation of the cause of the issues. You should, however, allow some flexibility as you may need to trial and adapt intervention strategies. For example, with John you could write:

"In collaboration with the school staff members, the following strategies will be trialled:

- At times when it is acceptable to the teacher, John will be able to write about his interest in Star Wars. He will be sensitively cued at other times by his teacher if he continues to talk inappropriately about this topic (questions, transitions).

- John will move to a different desk in the classroom so that he is closer to the front of the class to reduce distractions and have enough space to move his chair away from the table adequately (attends, positions).
- It will be negotiated with the teacher that some of the displays will be placed at the back of the classroom to support the children to keep focused on their work (attends).
- The occupational therapist will consult with the teacher about effective ways to support John to write words which he does not know how to spell (initiates, continues).
- The occupational therapist will also consult with the teacher about providing written instructions for the children at the outset of the task (initiates, continues)."

RE-EVALUATION FOR ENHANCED AND SATISFYING OCCUPATIONAL PERFORMANCE

Re-evaluation is considered in Chapter 13. The nature of re-evaluation or outcome measurement used depends on many factors, including what tools or indicators you have used during your assessment. *When* you write your report will influence *what* you write for this section. If you are writing your report at the time you are proposing your intervention plan, your re-evaluation will also be written as a plan (as neither have happened yet). For example, in John's report you could say:

"Plan for re-evaluation: At the end of the school term the occupational therapist plans to visit the school and review John's goal achievement through discussion with John, his teacher and parents."

You can also write an update to the report at a later stage, where you detail how the interventions went and to what extent the goals were achieved.

SIGNING AND DISTRIBUTING THE REPORT

Finally, you need to sign the report and consider to whom you will need to send copies. Your signature should be accompanied by your title (occupational therapy student) and counter-signed by a qualified therapist, if needed.

Consider who the report should be sent to and think about the permission you need to send the report to others. You may need to discuss this with the client and your educator to ensure that you are compliant with confidentiality policies. John's report, for example could include:

. . . . Date:. . . 12 June 2017. . . . .

Holly Johnson, third year occupational therapy student
Cc: parents, school, General Practitioner, occupational therapy file

FINAL CHECK WHEN WRITING PROGRESS NOTES AND REPORTS

Some important points to check when writing notes and reports are:

- Use a capital letter for the client's name and other names within the report. Ensure all names in the report are consistent (not copied and pasted incorrectly from another report).
- Check the language you use and how appropriate it is for the client and family to read, particularly in the interpretation section of the report.
- You may like to add elaborations to the report which help the flow of the writing, such as a summary of what the sections are going to cover (at the beginning) or what has been found (at the end).
- When writing clusters, firstly describe what was seen. As a separate step, consider a range of possibilities for why the performance was challenged. For example, if you say in the clusters that a person's challenge is organising himself and is due to the clutter on the work surface, then you are already deciding on the problem. You might miss other potential causes such as problems with concentration, etc.
- Look for consistency between the cluster, goal, interpretation of the cause and intervention. If you highlight an area of need and suggest that it is due to a reason, you should offer an intervention to address this challenge.
- You may offer more than one reason as potential causes of a challenge.
- An intervention may address multiple clusters.
- Check for any safety issues and ensure you have highlighted them in your clusters, interpretation and intervention plans.

CHAPTER SUMMARY

This chapter outlined the purpose of documentation and how it can support reasoning. We presented step-by-step guidance on completing two documentation styles, namely progress notes and reports. Both types of documentation require local contextualisation as there are many differing influences on the style, length and content of what is recorded. In any setting, however, the golden rules of making things clear for the client to understand and remaining focused on occupation apply.

APPENDIX 9.1

EXAMPLE REPORT

OCCUPATIONAL THERAPY REPORT

....

Date of report: 18/03/17   **Name of client:** Lee Bristol
Age: 27 years 2 months   **Date of birth:** 06/01/1990

BACKGROUND

INITIAL REFERRAL

Lee was referred to occupational therapy by his social worker Viktor Papir on 07/02/17, who expressed concern about Lee's self-care routines and specifically his diet and meal preparation. Lee has been living independently in a one-bedroom council property for the past three months since moving out from his parents' house in the next suburb.

Lee was diagnosed with Down's syndrome at birth. Lee works three days per week at a local supported employment service. Lee's parents prepare meals for him six nights a week in his flat and he eats at his parents' house every Sunday. Viktor has arranged for Lee to have a cleaner visit once a week and this has been working out well. Viktor is concerned about Lee's safety during meal preparation and his limited meal variety.

OCCUPATIONAL THERAPY ASSESSMENT

FOCUS FOR OCCUPATIONAL THERAPY ASSESSMENT

Occupational therapy is concerned with how people 'occupy' their time (i.e. their 'occupations'). The occupations we do impact on our health and well-being. Lee and his parents believe planning and cooking meals is important for Lee to live by himself and for his well-being. The occupational therapy assessment, therefore, observed Lee cooking a lunch of beans on toast with cheese.

OVERALL QUALITY OF PERFORMANCE DURING ASSESSMENT

Lee was socially appropriate whilst making his lunch. Lee did, however, display moderate physical effort and was markedly inefficient in his use of time, space and objects. He demonstrated a moderate level of risk of personal injury and environmental damage and required frequent assistance to successfully complete the task.

LEE'S SATISFACTION WITH HIS PERFORMANCE

Lee reports that he tries hard with cooking, although frequently loses track of what he is doing. He reports he would like more meal variety, as he tends to cook only a few dishes.

LEE'S PARENT'S SATISFACTION WITH HIS PERFORMANCE

Lee's parents would like him to be safe when he is cooking (they currently have concerns) and to increase the range of meals he prepares. Their own health concerns mean that they are not able to maintain the degree of support they currently provide.

SUMMARY OF HOME ENVIRONMENT AND OBJECTS

The kitchen in Lee's flat is compact and contains an electric cooker, oven, fridge and sink. There are cupboards above and below the small work surface. The cupboards contained a mixture of plates, bowls, mugs, pots and saucepans, with no clear order as to their location. The three drawers contained various cutlery, utensils, plastic bags, paper and other general items. Some of these were very close to the cooker and presented a risk. Lee used a tin opener with thin metal handles. The cheese grater was a flat metal surface with no handle.

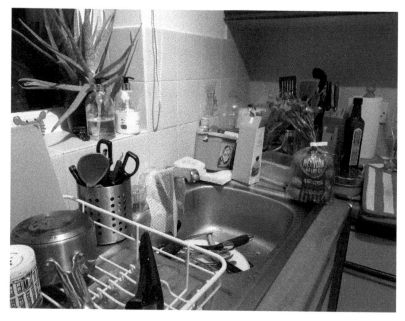

Figure 9.2 Picture of Lee's kitchen during assessment

SKILLS WHICH MOST IMPACTED ON PERFORMANCE

Lee was observed making his lunch and careful attention was given to his *social interaction, process and motor skills* as they impacted on his performance. Observations and potential reasons for Lee's challenges are listed in the following sections with recommendations described at the end of the report.

SOCIAL INTERACTION SKILLS

BEGINNING AND ENDING CONVERSATION

Lee could start and conclude conversations. His speech was clear as he conversed whilst making his lunch (approaches/starts, concludes/disengages, speaks fluently).

TALKING TOGETHER AND TAKING TURNS

On a few occasions, Lee asked for input from the occupational therapist and social worker, but he did not wait for a response to his question (replies, times response, times duration, takes turns).

Interpretation: Lee may have become distracted after he asked for assistance. As Lee has a learning difficulty associated with his diagnosis of Down's syndrome, it may be more challenging for him to do a task and listen/process instructions at the same time.

PROBLEM SOLVING WHEN ISSUES OCCURRED (SOCIAL INTERACTION)

Lee could ask for assistance during the task, but did not always wait for the answer to his question. These social interaction issues were minor and did not appear to impact significantly on Lee making his lunch (accommodates, benefits).

MOTOR SKILLS

CARRYING ITEMS

Lee could lift, move and transport items around the kitchen with no increased effort (moves, lifts, transports).

USING KITCHEN TOOLS

Lee's grip slipped while he was holding the cheese grater and using the tin opener. Lee did not press or squeeze the tip opener with enough force to use it to open the tin. He then used the knife to open the tin (grips, calibrates, manipulates, coordinates).

Interpretation: Lee's diagnosis of Down's syndrome means that he has had challenges with gripping and manipulating objects since childhood. The handles on the tin opener and the flat cheese grater with no handle also contributed to Lee's challenges.

PROCESS SKILLS

USING OBJECTS AND HANDLING THEM WITH CARE

Lee used a sharp knife to stab the tin to open it. This presented a safety concern. Lee also did not support the bread as he was buttering it, which caused it to move around on the chopping board (uses, handles).

Interpretation: The opener had small metal handles and was slippery to hold. Lee selected a knife to open the tin as an alternative. Lee did not appear to consider the safety risk of doing this, perhaps because he hasn't been made aware of these dangers.

STARTING ACTIONS, CONTINUING THEM IN A LOGICAL ORDER AND FINISHING

Lee frequently paused when buttering the bread and grating the cheese. Lee also used an illogical sequence, such as buttering the bread and then putting it in the toaster, and not turning on the hob when heating the beans. Lee continued to spread butter on his bread when it was completely covered and grated the whole 200g block of cheese (initiates, continues, sequences, terminates).

Interpretation: Lee may have forgotten the steps involved in making his lunch. Due to Lee's learning needs, he may have become mixed up in the sequencing of the task. Lee may not be aware of an appropriate portion of cheese to put on his beans.

GETTING ITEMS AND ORGANISING THEM

Lee placed items in random places and close to the edge of the work surface which meant they were in danger of being knocked to the floor (organises, gathers).

Interpretation: The crowded kitchen made it difficult to organise the items.

LOOKING FOR ITEMS AND PUTTING THEM AWAY WHEN FINISHED

Lee looked in a random way for the items he needed to make his lunch. He did not put any items away after he was finished with them (searches/locates, restores).

Interpretation: Lee's kitchen is cluttered without a clear place to put items. It may also be that Lee has not been expected to independently tidy his kitchen before, so he may not be aware of how to do this.

ADAPTATION SKILLS

SOLVING PROBLEMS AND DOING THINGS DIFFERENTLY

Lee did not notice that the beans were boiling rapidly and only when prompted did he take them off the heat and turn off the hob. He also did not notice that the newspapers were close to the hob and this presented a fire safety hazard (notices/responds, adjusts, accommodates, benefits).

Interpretation: Lee may not have remembered all the steps in the task. As he has only recently been living independently, he may not be aware of the potential safety hazards associated with cooking. His learning needs mean that this needs to be made more explicit and appropriately reinforced.

GOALS

LEE'S GOAL

"To live by myself and make my own food."

TARGETS/INTERVENTION OUTCOMES (DEVELOPED
WITH LEE AND THE OCCUPATIONAL THERAPIST)

– For Lee to safely and independently make beans on toast with cheese within three weeks.
– For Lee to safely make a meal of pasta and sauce for his family within six weeks.
– For Lee to add two more meals to his cooking repertoire and safely prepare them in 12 weeks.

RECOMMENDATIONS

Based on the assessment findings, the following strategies were collaboratively developed with Lee, his family and social worker. These will be trialled, modified and reviewed based on Lee's changing requirements and as per the plan for evaluation.

CHANGING TOOLS – LEE AND THE OCCUPATIONAL THERAPIST WILL SOURCE AND TRIAL

- A cheese grater which has a stable base and handle
- A tin opener with thicker handles and which requires less force to use
- Should this be unsuitable for Lee, then an electric can opener may be considered and training for Lee in how to use it will be required.
- Lee and his family may consider purchasing tins of beans with a ring pull lid, or plastic containers of beans.

ORGANISING THE KITCHEN – WITH ASSISTANCE FROM THE OCCUPATIONAL THERAPIST

- Lee will reorganise his kitchen cupboards and drawers so that related items are in one place.
- Drawers will be labelled in a way which will support Lee to remember where to put things.
- Lee will be encouraged to move non-kitchen items (such as DVDs, newspapers etc.) to a more appropriate space to create a clearer and safer workspace.
- The cleaner who visits Lee weekly will help maintain the organisation of his kitchen.

REMEMBERING STEPS IN COOKING – LEE AND THE OCCUPATIONAL THERAPIST

- Will make a series of cards with photos to show the steps in cooking.
- Will determine where these cards are stored so as not to add to the clutter in the kitchen.
- Will go through the cooking tasks multiple times so that Lee becomes familiar with the sequence using the cards.

PROMPTING LEE – PROBLEM SOLVING WITH THE OCCUPATIONAL THERAPIST

- A timer will be included in Lee's recipe sequence so that he is reminded to turn off the hob.
- Should this strategy prove insufficient, it may be suggested that Lee use a microwave to heat his beans.

PLAN FOR EVALUATION

Ongoing evaluation will occur as the occupational therapist continues to work with Lee on his cooking skills. This will involve regular discussions with Lee, his family and his social worker, along with observations by the occupational therapist. Lee's goals will be reviewed at the time-points specified in them. Comparisons between the initial and final occupational performance analysis will also be included in the evaluation.

Should you have any questions regarding this report, please contact Penny Door at The Occupational Therapy Department, telephone: 01234 567 890 or email: Penny.Door@ occupationaltherapy.com

Austin Davis   18/3/17   *Penny Door*   18/3/17

Austin Davis   Penny Door
Fourth year Occupational Therapy Student   Occupational Therapist

cc: Lee Bristol, social worker, General Practitioner, Lee's parents (with his permission), occupational therapy file

REFERENCES

Donaldson NA, McDermott A, Hollands K, Copley J, Davidson BJ (2004) 'Clinical reporting by occupational therapists and speech pathologists: Therapists' intentions and parental satisfaction'. *Advances in Speech-Language Pathology, 6*(1), 23–38.

Fisher AG (2009) *Occupational Therapy intervention process model: A model for planning and implementing top-down, client centred, and occupation-based interventions.* Fort Collins, CO: Three Star Press.

Groth-Marnat G, Horvath LS (2006) 'The psychological report: A review of current controversies'. *Journal of Clinical Psychology, 62*(1), 73–81.

Harvey VS (2006) 'Variables affecting the clarity of psychological reports'. *Journal of Clinical Psychology, 62*(1), 5–18.

Makepeace E, Zwicker JG (2014) 'Parent perspectives on occupational therapy assessment reports'. *British Journal of Occupational Therapy, 77*(11), 538–545.

Mastoras SM, Climie EA, McCrimmon AW, Schwean VL (2011) 'A CLEAR approach to report writing: A framework for improving the efficacy of psychoeducational reports'. *Canadian Journal of School Psychology, 26*(2), 127–147.

Royal College of Occupational Therapists (2015) *Code of ethics and professional conduct.* London, UK: Royal College of Occupational Therapists Ltd.

Simpson JM (1998) 'How good is your documentation?'. *British Journal of Occupational Therapy, 61*(10), 439.

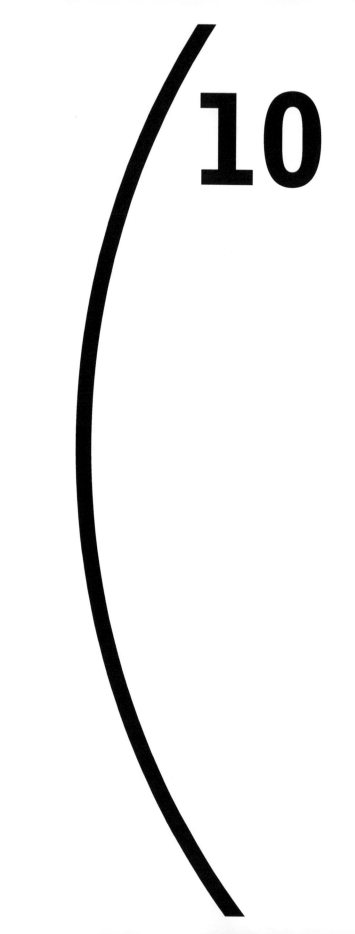

10

CHAPTER 10
ESTABLISHING, FINALISING OR REDEFINING CLIENT-CENTRED AND OCCUPATION-FOCUSED GOALS
Monica Moran and Karina Dancza

INTENDED CHAPTER OUTCOMES

By the end of this chapter, readers will have an overview of:

- How to write client-centred goals that are collaboratively developed by the therapist and the client
- The role of motivation in goal setting
- Strategies to deal with some common challenges of writing goals, such as understanding the difference between client-centred goals and therapy tasks, when priorities differ, and the difference between goals and intervention strategies
- Ideas on how student peers can help review one another's goals to become more competent in this area

STAGE IN THE OTIPM

As a reminder, your work is informed by practice models such as the Occupational Therapy Intervention Process Model (OTIPM; Fisher, 2009). This model provides you with a road map to plan and deliver your occupational therapy service, whatever the practice setting. In this chapter, we are focusing on goal setting. Please take a few moments to revisit the OTIPM diagram now to familiarise yourself with the concepts in this phase (Figure 10.1).

INTRODUCTION

In Chapter 7, you spent time getting to know your client's strengths and challenges so that you could select appropriate occupational therapy assessments. Now that you have more information about your client's performance capabilities, you are at the point of finalising goals with your client and/or his/her significant others in a format that allows you and your client to evaluate progress.

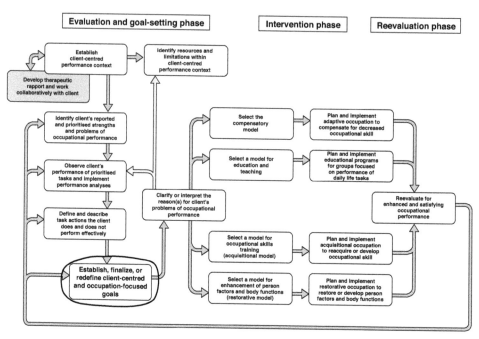

Figure 10.1 Schematic representation of the steps in the OTIPM: Establish, finalise or redefine client-centred and occupation-focused goals

Adapted from Fisher (2009). Available: www.innovativeotsolutions.com/content/wp-content/uploads/2014/01/English-OTIPM-handout.pdf. Reprinted with permission.

In addition, the articulation of client goals can enable you to demonstrate the effectiveness of your therapy interventions to the funders who support your service delivery (we will discuss service evaluation in more detail in Chapter 13).

The setting of goals with your client will relate to the prioritised occupations you have assessed. It may be that some of the details discussed in this chapter revisit what you have done in developing rapport and establishing the priority areas; that is fine. Although the occupational therapy process is presented in a linear way, there will be some going backwards and forwards.

BEING CLIENT-CENTRED AND THE ROLE OF CLIENT MOTIVATION

To be able to develop effective goals, it is vital that you can tap into the *hopes, dreams and aspirations of your clients*. Clients may have a global vision of what they want to achieve, for example:

"I want to get back to work."
"I want to have friends."

"I want to live independently at home."
"I want to be a good parent."
"I want to be happy."

Your role is to collaborate with your clients in the identification and setting of targets that move them towards their aspirations. When working with clients, there is compelling evidence to suggest that those who are engaged in the development of their own goals have a greater sense of ownership and take a more active role in their therapy (King and Ziviani, 2015). We can start to explore this relationship through considering *Self Determination Theory* (Ryan and Deci, 2008). This important theory has wide application to the process of collaborative goal setting. Three constructs are identified within Self Determination Theory:

1 **Relatedness**, acknowledging the importance of the therapeutic relationship between therapist and client
2 **Client autonomy**, reflecting the importance of involving the client in goal formulation
3 **A sense of client competence**, that the goals proposed are within the capacity of the client

When prioritising with a client what is important (as we did in Chapter 7), questions which relate to the three constructs within Self Determination Theory (Poulsen, Ziviani and Cuskelly, 2015, p. 34) might be as follows.

1 **Relatedness**: "Do I feel supported in pursuing this goal (not directed or coerced)?"
2 **Client autonomy**: "How important is this goal to me?"
3 **A sense of client competence**: "How do I feel about my current performance?"

When you have observed the priority occupations and are refining the goals, questions the client might be concerned with could include the following.

1 **Relatedness**: "Can I get help working out what to do?"
2 **Client autonomy**: "Do I really want this?"
3 **A sense of client competence**: "What is my next step? How will I do this?"

As you work with the client in the intervention phase (Chapter 12), questions may shift to the following.

1 **Relatedness**: "Can I talk to someone and adjust my goal plans, if I need to?"
2 **Client autonomy:** "What can I do to reach this goal?"
3 **A sense of client competence**: "How do I rate my progress so far?"

Each of these three dimensions impacts on a person's motivation to engage in therapy. If intervention is not going as well as you hoped, revisit these dimensions with the client to determine if changes are required.

Self Determination Theory may also be useful in understanding others' motivation to engage in the therapeutic process. Family members, carers or teachers can have a significant role in co-identifying goals and delivering interventions. Inviting families and significant others into the collaborative process provides them with a sense of ownership and competence in their capacity to continue with the implementation of the interventions after you finish your placement.

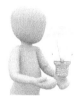

ACTIVITY

....

Using *Self Determination Theory* to help with goal setting, reflect on the following questions (King and Ziviani, 2015) in relation to the work you have been doing with clients on your placement.

RELATEDNESS

— Consider how you built your therapeutic relationships with clients and significant others. What impact do you think this had on how they prioritised their occupations?
— Think about ways in which you build trust with your clients. How do you demonstrate your understanding of their lived experience and how do you instil hope?

CLIENT AUTONOMY

— How can you promote autonomy for your clients in their goal setting (whilst being mindful of cultural diversity)? What opportunities have you created to promote choice, provide information regarding options and clarify concerns?

A SENSE OF CLIENT COMPETENCE

— What strategies do you use to support clients to identify goals that are congruent with their competence? Think about your activity analysis skills and ways you have learned to break down and pace activities (see Chapter 4).

TOOLS TO HELP IDENTIFY CLIENT PRIORITIES FOR GOAL SETTING

Client-centred collaborative goals *outline what it is that the client wants to do and will be able to do or achieve following intervention.* A range of resources are available for you to use with your clients to help identify and articulate their priorities and start developing goals for therapy. Your choice of tool will depend on the placement setting and performance context of the client.

A widely used example of an occupationally focused assessment to support goal setting is the *Canadian Occupational Performance Measure* (COPM; Law, Baptiste, Carswell-Opzoomer, McColl, Polatajko and Pollock, 1991). This interview tool guides you to explore and rank the importance of a person's self-care, productivity and leisure occupations.

A more general tool is *Goal Attainment Scaling* (GAS; Kiresuk and Sherman, 1968). It provides a common tool for goal identification across a variety of professions and enables you to measure progress through a five-point rating scale.

More specialist tools are available to assist in goal setting with specific populations. One example is the *Belief in Goal Self-Competence Scale* (BiGSS; Ziviani, Poulsen, Kotaniemi and Law, 2014). This tool is used with children to evaluate their confidence in pursuing their goals.

Several tools are available to you that rely on images to facilitate the goal identification and goal setting processes. For children or adults who find it helpful to use pictures to indicate preferences, *Talking Mats* (Murphy, 1998) is a useful tool for priority identification and goal setting. A widely used tool for older adults is the *Activity Card Sort* (Baum and Edwards, 2008). This tool uses an extensive series of pictures to generate discussion about former and current occupations as well as aspirations for engagement in future occupations.

You may find that a good *narrative interview* enables you to establish a therapeutic relationship with your client, so be sure to revisit your learning about communication micro-skills and interview techniques from your university learning (see also Powrie and Hemsley, 2015 and Chapters 6 and 11). You may have a template already available or have learned to use a narrative interview tool such as the *Occupational Performance History Interview II* (OPHI-II; Kielhofner et al., 2004). Further information on these and other tools can be found in Pollock, Missiuna and Jones (2017).

Whatever tool you use, remember the focus is on the occupational priorities of your client. Your role is to collaboratively identify how goals and associated priority occupations can be framed into targets. If the client is accessing other professionals simultaneously (such as a doctor, physiotherapist, teacher, psychologist etc.) you may also need to liaise with these colleagues to ensure the goals are based on what is important for the client. A few coordinated meaningful goals can be more effective than many discipline specific goals (this will be further described later in this chapter). Discuss the possibilities, strengths and challenges associated with these tools with your educator.

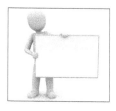

EDUCATOR EXAMPLES HERE:
GOAL-SETTING TOOLS

– Discuss with your student(s) and provide examples where available of goal setting
  tools and techniques used (or have the potential to be used) in this placement setting.
– Encourage students to look again at their university learning in relation to goal setting.

PERFORMANCE CONTEXTS

In developing goals, we cannot discount the impact of the environment. The environment in which your clients have grown up may inform what they see as possible for their future. If the environment has been restrictive, clients may not be able to envisage new possibilities. Part of your job may be to help your clients *see new possibilities for their future*.

Conversely your clients may currently be in an environment that they experience as more restrictive than they have previously occupied. They may be in a service environment that has priorities that are not aligned with what your clients want to achieve. For example, some acute services have priorities about rapid discharge that may not align with client goals of attaining levels of independent occupational performance prior to discharge. Ideally service providers and clients will have complementary priorities that reflect the human dignity for your client within the operational priorities of the organisation. As an occupational therapy student, you cannot change organisational priorities; but your awareness of potential conflicts between organisational priorities and client aspirations will allow you to support your clients in setting goals that best match the characteristics of their current situation, and also reflect future opportunities for participation.

ACTIVITY

What sort of environmental impacts have you noted that may influence your
client's capacity to set or achieve his/her goals? Make a note of them and use
this as a basis for discussion in supervision.

CONSIDERING CULTURE WHEN GOAL SETTING

As we discussed in Chapter 7, we find ourselves as occupational therapists working with people who may be different from ourselves in terms of their age, sexuality, religion, gender, belief systems and ethnicity. Understanding our own beliefs about participation and engagement in occupations based on our own upbringing, life experience and cultural background is an important first step to understanding the diversity and priorities of others.

One useful way to explore cultural differences and their impact on how people may respond to our services, is by understanding some of the characteristics of collectivist (high context) cultures and individualistic (low context) cultures (Masin, 2011). Collectivist cultures are characterised by a valuing of group/community relationships and goals, rather than an emphasis on individual goals that may be seen with people in individualistic cultures. For example, a woman recovering from a stroke who sees herself as belonging to a collectivist (high context) culture may articulate goals that focus on harmony within the family group. If she sees herself as belonging to an individualistic (low context) culture, she may prioritise goals that reflect her own attainment of autonomy in caring for herself. This difference was highlighted by a study of occupational therapy practice in Singapore. Yang, Shek, Tsunaka and Lim (2006, p. 182) stated that:

> Seven practitioners raised the issue of independence. They believed that it is important for clients to achieve independence in activities of daily living. However, they expressed difficulty applying this concept in the Singapore context due to three factors: client's values and beliefs about independence; social norms on care giving; and a profit driven society.

ACTIVITY

1   Revisit Chapter 7 and remind yourself of some of the examples of differences in priorities that you may encounter when working with people who are culturally different from yourself. Then consider the following questions:
    –   What strategies have you already covered in your university studies to prepare you for working with people of cultures different from your own?

- Are you familiar with the concepts of Cultural Sensitivity, Cultural Competence and Cultural Safety? What do they mean and how can you use these concepts to support your practice?
- What occupational therapy practice models are available to help you in your work with people from cultures different from your own?
- Who within your setting could help you gain a better understanding of the cultures of the people with whom you are working (if you are unfamiliar with them)?

2 You may wish to use your answers to these questions as a basis for a reflection or to update your learning objectives.

CONSIDERING CLIENT-CENTRED GOALS AND TARGETS

As discussed at the beginning of this chapter, a person's goals are based on what is motivating them and will determine what is possible to achieve from engagement with occupational therapy. They are personal and individual, such as "I want to get back to work" or "I want to be happy."

Rarely will goals be thought of by clients in a formulaic way, which tells us exactly what they want to achieve, how this will be measured and specified within a time frame. For example, "I will be able to get myself dressed safely and independently within three weeks." Specific targets for therapy can be helpful. These give us (and possibly clients too) an idea of what steps we can work on with them which will help them realise their goal.

Linking together the client-centred goal(s) with specific target(s) can help us understand what a client's *global goal might look like when it is achieved.* Table 10.1 provides an example of how a client-centred goal can be linked with targets.

Table 10.1 Client-centred goals and targets example

Client-centred goal	Targets
I want to get back to work as a TV presenter.	David will read from an auto-cue screen for 20 minutes within four weeks.
	David will conduct an eight-minute interview within six weeks.
	David will get himself ready (under one hour) to go out with occasional assistance within 12 weeks.

ACTIVITY
....

1   From the information you have previously gathered, answer the following
    questions:
    –   What is the client-centred goal(s) (i.e. be happy, live independently etc.)?
    –   How do the occupation(s) you assessed link with the client-centred goal(s)?
2   Use Table 10.1 to consider how to link the client-centred goals with targets.
    Targets need to be collaboratively developed with the client to ensure they
    reflect the goals, but your skills in activity and occupational performance
    analysis are important in supporting their development.
3   Could you use the same idea of goals and targets to frame your own
    placement learning objectives?

FORMATS FOR ARTICULATING CLIENT-CENTRED GOALS

There is no one correct format for writing goals. An essential element is the *collaborative development of the goal* so that your client agrees with the way forward and is invested in participating in the subsequent intervention or service delivered. In Table 10.1, we illustrated that a client-centred goal can be written in the client's own words and in a way which is meaningful for them. We have then suggested how these goals are used to guide our occupational therapy involvement. We have termed these steps *targets*, although some may call these sub-goals or shorter-term goals. For clarity, we will refer to:

–   **Goals** as the focus of a person's *hopes, dreams and aspirations*
–   **Targets** as the specific steps collaboratively developed to progress towards the goals

To help write these targets in a way which guides our therapy, you could frame them in a commonly used format: SMART. Each letter stands for a characteristic related to the goal formation. Over the years, the SMART acronym has been modified by various professional groups, so you may notice minor variations in the SMART format (King and Ziviani, 2015). The main elements are:

   S = Specific (being clear about what the client and therapist have decided they
      want to achieve, and relating this to the client-centred goal)
   M = Measurable (having a way of identifying how the client and therapist will
      estimate if the target is fully, partly or not achieved)
   A = Activity based (at the very least that the target includes activity that is a
      component of a necessary, valued and/or desired occupation for the client)

R = Realistic and relevant (for the life-course stage and performance capacity of the client, which can be particularly challenging to negotiate as there is an aspirational nature to goal setting and the client and therapist must retain hope for the attainment of the fullest possible performance capacity)

T = Timely or time bound (over what period will the client and therapist collaborate to achieve this target and goal and when will re-evaluation take place, resulting in another round of goal setting, modification of current goal or discharge from therapy if goals have been achieved)

ACTIVITY

1 Read through the example targets that follow and identify the SMART aspects of each.
   – Beth will collect her school dinner tray, sit down and eat her school dinner with her friends, by mid-September (three weeks).
   – Children in the year 3 playground will play cooperatively during lunch times to a level which is satisfactory to the teacher on duty, by the end of the Autumn term.
   – Children in the assembly hall will remain seated for the duration of the assembly, within four weeks.
   – Susan will complete four hours' work per day, three days a week by the end of July.
   – Frank will shave and wash himself in preparation for going to the day centre by 10am each weekday morning within five weeks (end of March).
   – By the end of week two, all members of the back-pain group will make themselves morning tea together.
2 Review your client's goals and think about writing targets in a way which is SMART. Collaboration with your client is essential, although as a novice you may need to spend some time yourself formulating targets in the SMART format.
3 Think about your own learning objectives. Review your own targets for the SMART format.

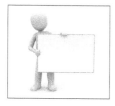

EDUCATOR EXAMPLES HERE: GOALS

– Provide students with example goals relevant for the placement setting and client(s).

DEVELOPING CLIENT-CENTRED GOALS IN A TEAM-BASED ENVIRONMENT

While on placement you will frequently find yourself working as part of an inter-professional or multidisciplinary team of service providers; they may be other health and social care professionals, educators or other vocational groups such as administrators. These colleagues will also have targets for your client. It is important to find out what processes exist to *share and discuss client goals* and how team members plan to enact them. Investigate if there are regular team meetings, case conferences or daily hand-overs in your placement facility. Try to get involved as appropriate and use the opportunity to find out what therapeutic goals are already in place for your client. This will also give you a chance to discuss the targets you have developed with your client and negotiate with your colleagues how these may be prioritised.

Table 10.2 provides an example of the multiple people in the team that may contribute to the goals and targets. Remember that the client and family members/significant others are part of the team.

Table 10.2 Operationalising person-centred goals – Judith with chronic back pain

Person-centred goals	Targets (SMART)	Indicative actions (what will be done and who will do it)
I want to do more with my partner and dogs.	**Walking the dogs:** Judith will join her partner and dogs for a 15-minute walk within three weeks.	– Before the first outing the occupational therapist will meet with Judith, her partner and the physiotherapist to plan her preferred route for a 15-minute dog walk. – Supported by the physiotherapist, Judith's partner will be encouraged to accompany her for short daily walks starting at five minutes per day and increasing to 10 minutes per day after one week. – Judith and her prescribing doctor will re-evaluate her medication regime to ensure that she is taking her pain relief medication at the optimum times for her planned increase in activity levels. – Judith will practice non-chemical pain management techniques (muscle relaxation and positive visualisation) guided by the occupational therapist, each day for one week as she increases her walking time. – The occupational therapist will refer Judith to a podiatrist to ensure that her footwear is providing her with adequate support for increased walking.

(Continued)

Table 10.2 (Continued)

	Driving to the coast: Judith will join her partner and dogs for an outing by car to the coast within one month.	– The occupational therapist will work with Judith to ensure that she is using safe transfer techniques to get in and out of the car. – The occupational therapist will assess Judith's sitting position in the car and assist with seating adjustments to ensure Judith is in a safe ergonomic posture. – Judith's partner will lift the dogs in and out of the car as they are large and would be too lively for Judith to transfer.
	Grooming the dogs: Judith will assist with weekly dog bathing and grooming within two months.	– Judith will work with the occupational therapist to complete a daily pain diary and identify when she is feeling most able to manage her pain and engage in activities. – Judith and her partner will work together to list the tasks involved in grooming the dogs and identify tasks she can do.
I want to get back to work.	Return to former work role: Judith will return to part-time work at her place of employment within five weeks.	– The occupational therapist will work with Judith and her employer to identify tasks she can complete in the workplace that will be within her pain and physical capacity. – The occupational therapist will work with Judith to practice strategies such as distraction and breathing techniques for managing pain in the workplace. – Judith will be introduced to the psychologist to trial some cognitive pain management techniques. – The occupational therapist will conduct a worksite visit and recommend environmental modifications to Judith's workstation to ensure optimum ergonomic fit.
	Re-develop work relationships: Judith will participate in work based meetings with her team within seven weeks.	– The occupational therapist will work with Judith and her supervisor to identify timing, duration, location and frequency of meetings, as well as Judith's expected contribution. Judith will prepare in advance for meetings including identifying her sitting and standing tolerances and communicating these requirements to her supervisor. – The psychologist will work with Judith on strategies she can use to be more confident and assertive in her role in the workplace.

DOCUMENTING YOUR GOALS

Chapter 9 described how you might document your involvement with a client. Once you have determined with your client and educator the goal(s) and targets, you will need to document these. This might be done in your progress notes and/or in your report.

A note of caution here. The goals and targets are what the client wishes to *do and will be able to do* following intervention. This can sometimes be confused with what *you* are planning on doing as an occupational therapy student. For example, it might be tempting to write:

 "To complete a handwriting assessment with David during his English lesson by week 4."

This is your plan for what *you* will do. This is not what your client will do by the end of your intervention. This could be included in the 'indicative actions' column as seen in Table 10.2. What might be achieved by the end of your intervention (and could be written as a target) is:

 "To write a half-page story in his English lesson by week 4."

Another common confusion for students is targets versus strategies. By keeping strategies separate, you can undertake many different strategies to meet a single target. For example, the *target* might be:

"For the children in the assembly hall to remain seated for assembly by the mid-term break."

Strategies for achieving this target might be:

"For children to be allowed to sit on chairs during assembly"
"For the assembly to involve a movement break after 15 minutes of seated time"

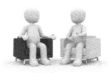

ACTIVITY
....

1 Together with a peer (if possible), review how you are writing the goals, targets and indicative actions by using these questions:
  – Is the goal what the person wishes for him-/herself?
  – Are targets written in a way which states what the *client* will achieve?
  – Are targets written in collaboration with the client/family/relevant setting staff?

- Do targets relate to occupation?
- Are targets SMART?

2   Use your notes as the basis of a reflection. In addition, consider:
  - How have you managed to honour your clients' hopes, dreams and aspirations for the future?
  - Have you experienced any ambivalence regarding your priorities and your clients' priorities?
  - How have you collaborated with other team members to ensure that the targets are harmonised? Could the client be overwhelmed, confused or conflicted?
  - How might you use these experiences of client-centred goal setting to inform your learning objectives for this placement and your ongoing competency development?

CHAPTER SUMMARY

This chapter outlined how Self Determination Theory (Ryan and Deci, 2008) can be used to understand a client's motivation for therapy and how this might influence clients' goals. It then explored how to negotiate client-centred goals and convert those goals into a format that allows planning and evaluations of interventions. Remember that client goals are often very broad and aspirational. Taking time with your clients to genuinely understand their goals and how they are framed by cultural, social and environmental milieu will be invaluable for the next step in the therapeutic process.

REFERENCES

Baum C, Edwards D (2008) *Activity card sort*. 2nd edn. Bethesda, MD: American Occupational Therapy Association Press.

Fisher AG (2009) *Occupational Therapy intervention process model: A model for planning and implementing top-down, client centred, and occupation-based interventions*. Fort Collins, CO: Three Star Press.

Kielhofner G, Mallinson T, Crawford C, Nowak M, Rigby M, Henry A, Walens D (2004) *A User's Manual for the OPHI-II: The occupational performance history interview-II (OPHI-II)*. Chicago: Model of Human Occupation Clearinghouse.

King G, Ziviani J (2015) 'What does engagement look like? Goal-directed behavior in therapy'. In AA Poulsen, J Ziviani, M Cuskelly (Ed.), *Goal setting and motivation in therapy: engaging children and parents*. London, UK, Jessica Kingsley Publishers, pp. 70–79.

Kiresuk TJ, Sherman RE (1968) 'Goal attainment scaling: A general method for evaluating comprehensive community mental health programs'. *Community Mental Health Journal*, 4(6), 443–453.

Law M, Baptiste S, Carswell-Opzoomer A, McColl MA, Polatajko H, Pollock N (1991) *Canadian occupational performance measure*. Toronto, ON: Canadian Association of Occupational Therapy Publications.

Masin HL (2011) 'Communicating with cultural sensitivity'. In: CM Davis, GM Musolino, eds, *Patient practitioner interaction: An experiential manual*. Thorofare, NJ: Slack Incorporated, pp. 143–156.

Murphy J (1998) 'Talking mats: Speech and language research in practice'. *Speech and Language Therapy in Practice*, Autumn, 11–14. Available: www.talkingmats.com [June 22, 2017].

Pollock N, Missiuna C, Jones J (2017) 'Occupational goal setting with children and families'. In: S Rodger, A Kennedy-Behr, eds, *Occupation-centred practice with children: A practical guide for occupational therapists*. 2nd edn. West Sussex, UK: Wiley-Blackwell, pp. 91–110.

Poulsen A, Ziviani J, Cuskelly M (2015) 'The science of goal setting'. In: A Poulsen, J Ziviani, M Cuskelly, eds, *Goal setting and motivation in therapy – Engaging children and parents*. London: Jessica Kingsley Publications, pp. 28–39.

Powrie B, Hemsley B (2015) 'Goal identification when communication is a challenge'. In: A Poulsen, J Ziviani, M Cuskelly, eds, *Goal setting and motivation in therapy: Engaging children and parents*. London: Jessica Kingsley Publishers, pp. 131–142.

Ryan RM, Deci EL (2008) 'A self-determination theory approach to psychotherapy: The motivational basis for effective change'. *Canadian Psychology*, 49(3), 186–193.

Yang S, Shek MP, Tsunaka M, Lim HB (2006) 'Cultural influences on occupational therapy practice in Singapore: A pilot study'. *Occupational Therapy International*, 13(3), 176–192.

Ziviani J, Poulsen AA, Kotaniemi K, Law M (2014) 'The Belief in Goal Self-Competence Scale (BiGSS) – Exploring a new way to support individual goal pursuit and document occupational therapy outcomes in paediatric practice'. *Australian Occupational Therapy Journal*, 61(5), 316–324.

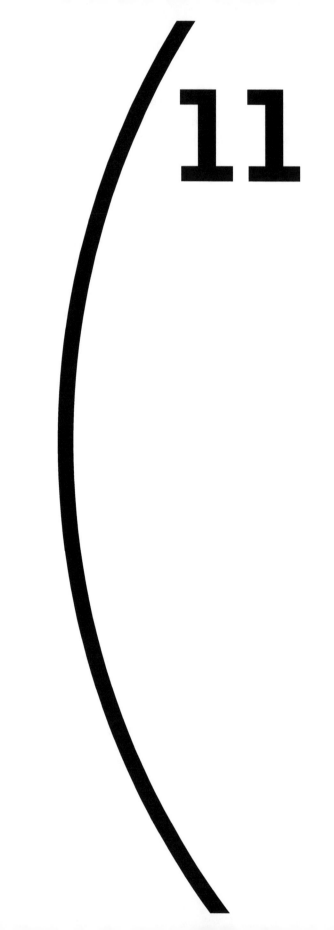

11

CHAPTER 11
CLARIFYING OR INTERPRETING THE REASON(S) FOR CLIENT'S PROBLEMS OF OCCUPATIONAL PERFORMANCE
Anita Volkert and Karina Dancza

INTENDED CHAPTER OUTCOMES

By the end of this chapter, readers will have an overview of:

- A step-by-step approach to identifying challenges in occupational performance and generating a range of ideas about those challenges
- The importance of making professional reasoning decisions transparent and linked to intervention opportunities
- Guidance for educators in supporting the development of students' reasoning through supervision

STAGE IN THE OTIPM

In this book, we have been following the Occupational Therapy Intervention Process Model (OTIPM; Fisher, 2009) to guide practice. This chapter will explore one of the critical features of the OTIPM: the step that encourages you to stop and think about your reasoning so you can plan appropriate interventions (Figure 11.1).

INTRODUCTION

A critical phase in the occupational therapy process, and one which is often not clear to students, is how to determine from the assessment information the potential reasons why a person is having difficulty performing his/her occupations. Within the OTIPM, there is a specific step leading the therapist to "Clarify or interpret the reason(s) for client's problems of occupational performance." This encourages us to pause and thoroughly consider the range of possible reasons for challenges in occupational performance. Clarity in our reasoning will enable us to defend our judgements and offer reasonable justification for our interventions. It also encourages us to think broadly and be creative in our intervention approaches.

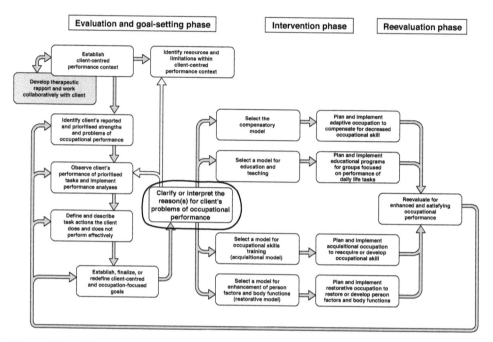

Figure 11.1 Schematic representation of the steps in the OTIPM: Clarify or interpret the reason(s) for client's problems of occupational performance

Adapted from Fisher (2009). Available: www.innovativeotsolutions.com/content/wp-content/uploads/2014/01/English-OTIPM-handout.pdf. Reprinted with permission.

This chapter will explore ways of making decisions transparent. We will link our occupational performance analysis results (from Chapter 8) and clusters created (from Chapter 9) with potential reasons for challenges with occupational performance. These reasons will form the basis of our intervention. Common pitfalls for students and educators will be highlighted, with suggestions for how to address these through supervision, action and reflection.

THE 'HIDDEN' NATURE OF REASONING

Expert practitioners appear to be able to make quick decisions based on the situation at hand, without articulating precisely how they made that decision (Eraut, 2004, 2007). Therefore, reasoning can appear *hidden*. Taking time to pause and clarify the potential causes of occupational performance issues using reasoning types can help you to understand and unpack why decisions might be made.

"Clarifying or interpreting the reason(s) for client's problems of occupational performance" can also be described as *professional reasoning* (Schell and Schell, 2008). The process of reasoning is often difficult to articulate. That makes it complicated to teach and to learn (Unsworth and Baker, 2016). Describing our reasoning is, however, worth our time and effort as it helps us explain our approach to clients, supervisors and team members, and can offer clarity for ourselves. It can also help us justify why a qualified occupational therapist is needed within a service, as well as identify, measure and potentially research the outcomes we achieve.

There is a variety of approaches to professional reasoning, and at least eight types of reasoning are described by Schell and Schell (2008): scientific, diagnostic, procedural, narrative, pragmatic, ethical, interactive and conditional. Table 11.1 provides a very brief summary of these professional reasoning types, and you are encouraged to read about these more widely and use this in your supervision discussions.

You might be asking yourself at this stage, what is the point of knowing about reasoning types? They can seem like abstract concepts. You may not even be consciously aware of which type of reasoning you are using at the point you make decisions. Using different types of reasoning to unpack decision making may, however, help you reflect on your own knowledge and skills. This can also help you understand people's different priorities.

For example, Chapter 7 introduced *interactive reasoning* as useful when you are negotiating priority areas for your involvement. By thinking about how you conducted conversations with clients and others, you may decide that interactive reasoning is something you want to develop further.

Another example might be that if on reflection you consider your knowledge of a person's diagnosis and its impact on occupational performance is insufficient (i.e. *conditional reasoning*), you may decide to make this a focus for your future learning.

Table 11.1 Reasoning types (Schell and Schell, 2008)

Reasoning type	Description
Scientific	Systematically creating, testing and using knowledge to make decisions
Diagnostic	Using the occupational therapy process to understand occupational performance challenges and infer a cause to make an occupational therapy diagnosis
Narrative	Decision making based on analysing stories of people's lives to understand the person as an occupational being
Ethical	Thinking and acting based on moral and ethical imperatives
Interactive	Building relationships to make decisions through understanding the person and their life context
Conditional	Using knowledge of a condition to predict a future situation for the person
Procedural	Rule-based decision making
Pragmatic	Decision making based on practical contextual factors which facilitate or inhibit occupation

At times, you may find that what you want to do does not match the service or others' expectations. For example, you might wish to understand a person's story (using *narrative reasoning*), but the service is provided in a fast-paced hospital setting where decisions are made based primarily on resources (requiring *pragmatic reasoning*) and medical diagnosis (requiring *conditional reasoning*). Exploring decision making through the lens of reasoning types may offer some clarity to these competing demands.

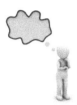

ACTIVITY
....

Think about a situation in a previous placement where a decision was made. **What types of reasoning do you think were being used to make those decisions?** Remember that it is likely that multiple types of reasoning will be used to guide decision making at any one time. For example:

–   In an acute hospital ward, where the focus is on discharging people home, you might use *conditional reasoning* (i.e. knowledge of the client's condition to guide your decisions), *procedural reasoning* (i.e. knowledge of the hospital processes to guide decisions) and *pragmatic reasoning* (i.e. knowledge of available resources to guide decisions).
–   In a community mental health team, you might use *narrative reasoning* (i.e. knowledge of the person's story to guide decisions) and *diagnostic reasoning* (i.e. knowledge of how the occupational performance is challenged to guide decisions).

LINKING ASSESSMENT FINDINGS WITH REASONING

The OTIPM encourages us to carefully consider what we have found out from our assessments and reason what might be causing the occupational performance challenges. This could be considered a form of *diagnostic reasoning*. While there are other ways to articulate your reasoning (as we have described), we will take you through this process step-by-step, to maintain coherence with the occupational therapy process presented in the OTIPM.

As occupational therapists, we need to allow ourselves *time to generate* (or formulate) our ideas about potential causes of occupational performance problems. These initial ideas often require refinement through conversations with clients, more experienced colleagues and others. We also learn a lot from trialling ideas, adjusting things as we work with clients and reflecting on the outcomes.

As a starting point for this process, think about our occupational therapy theory. This tells us that occupational performance is a combination of the person's abilities and previous experience, combined with the task's challenge and the environmental context (Law, Cooper, Strong, Stewart, Rigby and Letts, 1996). Therefore, there are likely to be *multiple factors* which are challenging the occupational performance. Make sure you *keep an open mind* to all possibilities, rather than determining one factor and then attributing all the problems to that one cause.

For example, if a child is pressing too softly on the paper when writing so that no marks can be seen (potentially seen as 'calibrates' on the occupational performance analysis template, as described in Chapters 4 and 8), this problem could be attributed to any of the following:

- The child has a weak grip on the pencil.
- Having a single sheet of paper on the table makes the surface too hard.
- The chair is too low, preventing the child from pressing down sufficiently on the paper.
- The pencil lead is too hard.
- The child has never used a pencil before, etc.

The reason for defining the cause is so that intervention can be appropriately targeted. In the previous example, if you thought the cause was that the child had never used a pencil before, the intervention would likely be increased exposure, practice and demonstration. However, if you thought the cause was the chair height and the child's low position at the table, you would change something about the chair and table. Table 11.2 illustrates links between potential causes of occupational performance challenges and interventions.

Table 11.2 Examples of potential causes and the link with interventions

Possible cause	Intervention suggestion
The child has a weak grip on the pencil.	Provide a thicker pencil or suitable pencil grip.
Having a single sheet of paper on the table makes the surface too hard.	Provide a pad of paper for the child.
The chair is too low, preventing the child from pressing down sufficiently on the paper.	Provide a higher chair or lower table.
The pencil lead is too hard.	Replace the pencil with a softer pencil or a felt pen.
The child has never used a pencil before.	Provide opportunities for instruction and practice with a range of writing implements (pencils, felt pens, crayons etc.).

The following sections take you through three steps to help you consider potential causes of the occupational performance challenges you observed during your occupational performance analysis.

STEP 1 FOR STUDENTS: BLUE-SKY THINKING

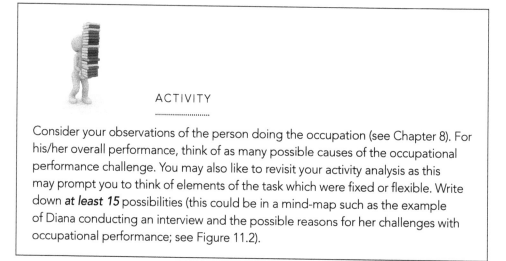

ACTIVITY

....

Consider your observations of the person doing the occupation (see Chapter 8). For his/her overall performance, think of as many possible causes of the occupational performance challenge. You may also like to revisit your activity analysis as this may prompt you to think of elements of the task which were fixed or flexible. Write down *at least 15* possibilities (this could be in a mind-map such as the example of Diana conducting an interview and the possible reasons for her challenges with occupational performance; see Figure 11.2).

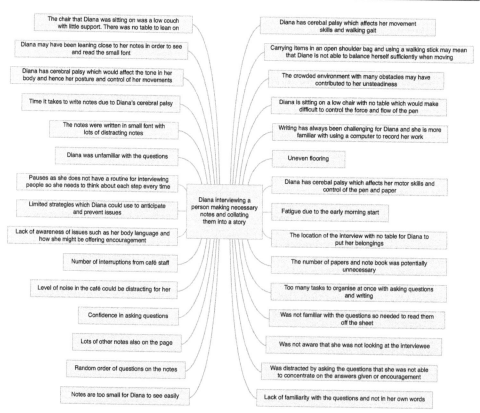

Figure 11.2 Mind map for blue sky thinking

STEP 2 FOR STUDENTS: REVISIT YOUR CLUSTERS

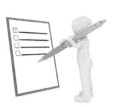

ACTIVITY

Look at the clusters you created within your report (see Chapter 9). For each cluster, list the possible causes for that specific cluster (you can select from your blue-sky list and add others). Table 11.3 offers an illustration of how this was done using the mind map example of Diana conducting an interview.

Table 11.3 Example of clusters and possible causes

Cluster	Possible causes . . .
Speaks fluently, questions, times response, times duration Diana spoke in a hesitant manner with frequent short pauses. She left some responses 'hanging in the air' as she looked at her question sheet, which disrupted the conversation. Diana delayed asking the questions and responding to the interviewee's answers, which further disrupted the social interaction. She also asked questions which she had previously asked, resulting in her supervisor asking some of the questions.	– Lack of familiarity with the questions and not in her own words – Notes are too small for Diana to see easily – Random order of questions on the notes – Lots of other notes on the page – Confidence in asking questions – Level of noise in the café could be distracting for her – Number of interruptions from café staff
Initiates, continues, heeds, terminates Diana hesitated before sitting down, paused before she retrieved her paper, notebook and pen and paused between asking questions. Diana also paused in the middle of asking questions, writing something, then returning to asking the question. Diana stopped the interview before all the questions were asked and the supervisor took over the interview.	– No routine for interviewing people, so Diana needs to think about each step every time – Lack of familiarity with the questions – Notes were written in small font with lots of distracting notes – The time it takes to write notes due to Diana's cerebral palsy – Fatigue due to the early morning start

ACTIVITY
....

From your blue-sky thinking, how many potential causes did you use in your cluster-potential cause lists? What didn't you use? Why was this? Note these down as points to discuss with your educator.

STEP 3 FOR STUDENTS: MODELS OF OCCUPATIONAL THERAPY

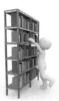

ACTIVITY
....

Revisit the Models of Occupational Therapy (see Chapter 3). Consider:
–   Which of your possibilities for the cause(s) of occupational performance challenges fit within the constructs addressed by these models? For example, do any relate to volition, habituation or performance capacity as described by Kielhofner (2008)?
–   How do the models prompt you to think about other causes? Note any other potential causes you have identified under each cluster.

GUIDANCE FOR EDUCATORS WITHIN SUPERVISION DISCUSSIONS

For students to develop their professional reasoning skills, it is vital that there are opportunities to discuss ideas, and that students are appropriately challenged to advance those ideas (Unsworth and Baker, 2016). This section will describe a structure and some prompts which may help guide you as an educator to enable students' exploration of professional reasoning. Students reading this section may also like to reflect on the question prompts to advance their thinking in preparation for these discussions in supervision.

It is likely that these discussions will need to be revisited during the placement as ideas may be formulated initially, but students will need space and time to try them out to consolidate their learning (also discussed in Chapter 14).

OPENING THE SUPERVISION DISCUSSION
Begin with a general debrief of the week, answering any urgent questions. Following this, you could focus on the preparation tasks which have been described for students to complete (Steps 1–3 listed earlier). To explore how they got on with this, you might ask:

"What do you think was the point of this task?"

"How did you find it?"

"What was easy or difficult about it? Why?"

These questions can help you to get a sense of how excited or unenthused students were about the task. Using reflective listening strategies (i.e. "so you found the task quite challenging . . .") can help you and the students explore the complexity associated with reasoning.

PROGRESSING THE SUPERVISION DISCUSSION
The focus now shifts to the specifics of reasoning. Each step outlined for the students will be discussed in turn, with prompt questions for you as educator to facilitate discussions.

STEP 1, SUPERVISION DISCUSSION: BLUE-SKY THINKING
Blue-sky thinking is intended to encourage students to think widely about what is happening. Questions which might help these discussions include:

"Tell me about your blue sky thinking. What possibilities do you think were 'out there' or unpredictable?"

"What possibilities were common place or predictable?"

"Why do you say that?"

Look for the possibilities which were *unpredictable* and those which *generated new thinking*. Blue-sky thinking encourages analysis of each situation individually, rather than seeing the same causes for each problem encountered.

If students did not create a wide list, then perhaps they are being too restrictive in their ideas about what is causing the challenges (i.e. attributing everything to a diagnosis and not considering wider factors such as the environment, the motivation of the person, previous experiences etc.). Exploring together with students using prompt questions about what was happening (considering the person, environment and occupation) can be helpful here. Also, highlighting how their activity analysis can also help them identify possible elements which may have contributed can also be useful. Reassure them that at this stage there are no 'wrong' or 'stupid' ideas. You could ask:

"What are the risks of thinking it is the same cause for every problem?"
"What do you think might happen if we think differently?"
"What might be another way of doing this?"
"In what other situations might you use this technique again?"
"Have you seen anyone else using this technique?"

These questions help to highlight how reasoning is part of what is required as a professional. This is not unique to occupational therapy, and students may have experienced other professionals engaging with similar reasoning processes. If they haven't, it could prompt them to seek out and ask other professionals (including other occupational therapists) about their reasoning. Support students to recognise that their reasoning can be enhanced through inter-professional deliberations.

STEP 2, SUPERVISION DISCUSSION: REVISIT YOUR CLUSTERS
This step in the decision-making process is designed to reinforce to students that as qualified professionals, they need to be able to analyse new situations, reason, then justify their decisions. Following a 'recipe' for therapy would be what was expected of an unqualified person. Explore with the students how to make the links between the clusters they created and potential causes of these challenges, with questions such as:

> "How did you link your blue-sky thinking to your clusters?"
> "Did they all fit?"
> "Tell me about your thinking in relation to how you made your decisions."
> "For the ones which didn't fit your clusters, what do you think about that?"
> "Is there another way of looking at this?"

These questions help students to decide what possibilities are viable and useful, and which ones need to be set aside. This is the first phase of a filtering process. Part of the discussions will need to be around what you as an educator think is possible within the placement context. Be careful, however, not to limit ideas unnecessarily because of historical processes (i.e. excluding something because of the way it has always been done).

You may wish to take a calculated risk with the students' ideas. Learning can be enhanced when students try out their ideas and learn from their successes and mistakes (discussed further in Chapter 14). If students have some ideas which you suspect might not work, but they won't cause any harm to try out, then you could allow them to find out for themselves through having a go and reporting back on the pros and cons of their idea.

STEP 3, SUPERVISION DISCUSSION: MODELS OF
OCCUPATIONAL THERAPY
Step 3 was designed to help students to link their ideas to models of occupational therapy. This makes explicit the relevance of theory and it can help broaden their ideas and think systematically about reasoning. Using Chapter 3 or the model diagrams as prompts, work together with students and share ideas about how to use models to better understand the occupational challenges of the clients with whom they are currently working, such as:

> "What happened when you used a model?"
> "What do you think caused that to happen? Why?"
> "What assumptions had you made about the causes of the occupational
>   performance challenges? How were these assumptions verified or disproven?"
> "What other ideas did looking at the models generate?"

"How did your thinking change when you used a model?"
"What other tools might help you think about this (such as the International
    Classification of Functioning, Disability and Health)?"

CONCLUDING THE SUPERVISION DISCUSSION

Congratulating the students for their efforts acknowledges the challenging nature of
reasoning and can encourage them to continue to develop this essential skill. Reinforcing
the process they have used, where they devised a range of possibilities and refined them
through using the clusters and models of practice, can help students reflect on how their
thinking about this situation has developed.

These discussions can help you check that the students are able to link their reasoning
with their clusters and models of practice. This could be an important part of the
assessment of the students' placement competencies. If the students have not been able to
do the preparation, then you may wish to work through some examples together to model
how you as an expert undertake this reasoning process.

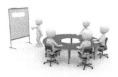

ACTIVITY
....

As a summary activity, you could ask students to present the arguments they
have developed about the potential cause(s) of the occupational performance
issues to yourself or a peer for comment. This argument needs to be convincing
and use evidence from the observations, and possibly from the literature, to back
up suggestions.

ADVICE FOR STUDENTS: WHAT IF THE REASONING PROCESS IS STILL UNCLEAR?

The reasoning process should highlight some potential causes for occupational performance
challenges. In many cases, this is enough to make a start on planning and implementing
interventions. In some cases, however, you will need to gather further information. The
first thing to do is to think about what you need to find out and why. You need to have a
clear rationale for undertaking more assessments: remember, an assessment can be stressful
for the person and it is also time-consuming for you and the client.

Once your rationale is clear, consider what might help you to gather this further information:

- Conduct another observation of the same occupation.
- Observe a different occupation for comparison.

- Conduct other assessments which are standardised or non-standardised. These might focus on the environment, task or person (e.g. body function/structure tests, environmental analysis, seating assessment). Think about the assessments you have been introduced to at university or on previous placements. Also, speak with your educator about the options available and suitability of these.
- Use a different occupational therapy model or frame of reference to consider different perspectives.
- Liaise with other professionals either within the setting or wider team, as the challenges may be better understood from a different professional's perspective.

A NOTE OF CAUTION . . .

Sometimes you as a student might feel a bit 'stuck' in this thinking phase. You may be worried about testing out some of your ideas in practice without having all your questions answered. You will be guided by your educator, but it is also useful to try out some intervention ideas and see what difference they make. You will be constantly assessing, even during the intervention phase, to maximise the effectiveness of the intervention. You cannot predict what will happen until you try it out!

DOCUMENTING YOUR UNDERSTANDING OF THE CAUSE OF OCCUPATIONAL PERFORMANCE CHALLENGES

Remember that you need to summarise your interpretations in the occupational therapy notes and report. Keep in mind that *your interpretations of the cause(s) are systematically and logically thought through estimates*; part of the 'art' of occupational therapy is to use the information available and trial interventions based on these estimates. Have a look again at Chapter 9 for examples of how to write your interpretation(s) of causes under each cluster.

ACTIVITY

1   Update your report with your ideas about the potential cause(s) of the occupational performance challenges.
2   Consider using the activities in this chapter as the basis of a reflection. How might you include this to inform your learning objectives?

CHAPTER SUMMARY

Determining from assessment information the potential reasons why a person is having difficulty performing his/her occupations is a crucial step within the occupational therapy process. Within the OTIPM, there is a specific step leading the therapist to "Clarify or interpret the reason(s) for client's problems of occupational performance." This step assists the student or qualified occupational therapist to identify challenges in occupational performance and generate a range of ideas about those challenges. Notions of professional reasoning discussed in this chapter enable us to think broadly and creatively, and offer justification for our interventions.

REFERENCES

Eraut M (2004) 'The practice of reflection'. *Learning in Health and Social Care, 3,* 47–52.

Eraut M (2007) 'Learning from other people in the workplace'. *Oxford Review of Education, 33*(4), 403–422.

Fisher AG (2009) *Occupational therapy intervention process model: A model for planning and implementing top-down, client centred, and occupation-based interventions.* Fort Collins, CO: Three Star Press.

Kielhofner G (2008) *A model of human occupation: Theory and application.* 4th edn. Baltimore, MD: Lippincott Williams & Wilkins.

Law M, Cooper B, Strong S, Stewart D, Rigby P, Letts L (1996) 'The Person-Environment-Occupational Model: A transactive approach to occupational performance'. *Canadian Journal of Occupational Therapy, 63*(1), 9–23.

Schell BAB, Schell JW, eds (2008) *Clinical and professional reasoning in occupational therapy.* Philadelphia, PA: Walters Kluwer/Lippincott, Williams & Wilkins.

Unsworth CA, Baker A (2016) 'A systematic review of professional reasoning literature in occupational therapy'. *British Journal of Occupational Therapy, 79*(1), 5–16.

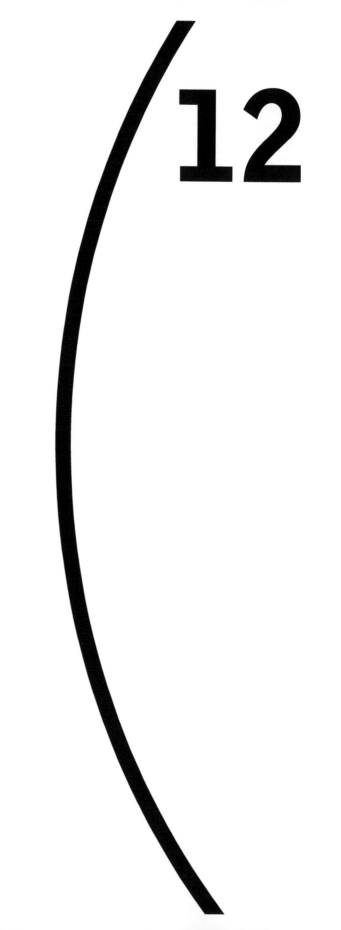

12

CHAPTER 12
INTERVENTION PHASE
Sue Mesa and Karina Dancza

INTENDED CHAPTER OUTCOMES

By the end of this chapter, readers will have an overview of:

- The types of interventions that are outlined in the OTIPM
- How intervention can be delivered on an individual, group or community basis
- How to use your assessment findings to justify your choice of intervention
- How you might draw on theories from outside of occupational therapy to support your intervention, but keep these within an occupation-centred approach
- What to consider when carrying out an intervention plan
- How to gain feedback on your performance

STAGE IN THE OTIPM

This chapter presents the intervention phase within the Occupational Therapy Intervention Process Model (OTIPM; Fisher, 2009). The OTIPM considers interventions under four broad intervention headings (Figure 12.1). Once an intervention category has been chosen, the next stage is to plan and carry out the intervention. Reflect on your progress to date using the OTIPM diagram in preparation for the detail explored in this chapter.

INTRODUCTION

There are many ways of enabling a person to do their occupations. This chapter will help you to use your assessment findings and professional reasoning to plan and carry out your interventions. The OTIPM invites you to think about the main purpose of your intervention:

1 To *compensate* (e.g. change the way an occupation is done, use equipment, modify the physical/social environment)
2 To *educate* (e.g. run workshops or lectures to groups which are related to occupational performance)
3 To *develop skills* (e.g. restore, develop, enhance or prevent loss of skills)
4 To *enhance body functions/person factors* (e.g. using occupations with the aim of changing something about a person's body)

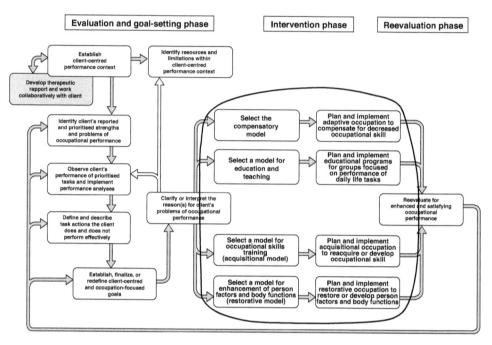

Figure 12.1 Schematic representation of the steps in the OTIPM – Intervention phase

Adapted from Fisher (2009). Available: www.innovativeotsolutions.com/content/wp-content/uploads/2014/01/English-OTIPM-handout.pdf. Reprinted with permission.

As we work through this chapter, you may think that intervention ideas could fit into more than one of these 'categories'. That is fine. What makes them useful is how they help us consider our *primary intention* for the intervention.

INDIVIDUAL, GROUP OR COMMUNITY INTERVENTION APPROACHES

Historically, occupational therapy has predominantly focused on individual clients (Case-Smith and Arbesman, 2008). There is, however, an argument that working with groups and communities using health promotion and prevention strategies is one of the most cost-effective interventions for improving health and well-being (World Health Organisation, 2015).

Figure 12.2 outlines how occupational therapy can be delivered through a graduated approach, where appropriate interventions are offered universally (the base of the triangle) with the intention of addressing most needs. Where more specific provision is required to meet the needs of a group of people, a targeted group approach is used. Finally, the most intensive, individual interventions are limited to those people for whom universal and

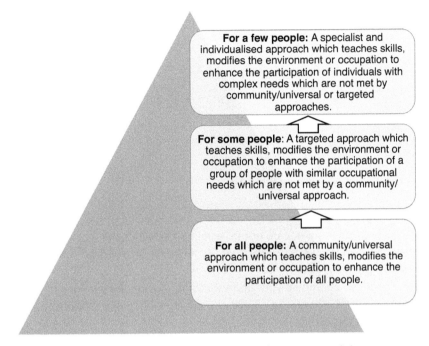

Figure 12.2 A graduated approach to the delivery of occupational therapy services
Adapted from Missiuna et al. (2012) and Dancza (2015).

targeted approaches are insufficient. The Canadian school-based occupational therapy research project *Partnering for Change* (Missiuna et al., 2012) is an example of this graduated approach to occupational therapy service delivery.

When you are working with a client through the OTIPM, the focus is on working with individual clients. To help you consider how you might use the information you have gathered to develop a group or community intervention plan, the *Classroom Intervention Reasoning Approach* (Dancza, Missiuna and Pollock, 2017) was developed. This approach outlines two ways of structuring the decision-making process for whole class or whole school interventions (although it could be applied to any groups or communities):

1 An intervention for an individual can be used with a group or community experiencing similar needs.
2 A group or community's needs are identified through observations of multiple clients, combining the data and using it to design suitable group interventions.

What is important in individual, group or community interventions is that you can demonstrate your professional reasoning and clearly link your assessment findings to your preferred intervention options. Remember that you are accountable as a professional for the suggestions you make.

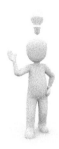

ACTIVITY
....

Think about your assessment information.

- Was the priority for the setting an individual or specific group activity or time of day (e.g. lunchtimes, care home recreation activities etc.)?
- How might an intervention you have identified for an individual be applied to a wider group?
- How might you combine your understanding of your observations of different people whilst they were doing this one activity? What intervention(s) could be trialled with this group?

In the following sections, we describe the intervention approaches suggested in the OTIPM in more depth. We offer examples of a graduated approach to intervention within each section.

SELECT A COMPENSATORY MODEL: PLAN AND IMPLEMENT ADAPTIVE OCCUPATION TO COMPENSATE FOR DECREASED OCCUPATIONAL SKILL

The focus of this intervention approach is to *compensate* for difficulties and find a way around a person's challenges. You can do this by:

- Teaching the person new ways of doing things to make them easier (e.g. teaching someone to dress with one hand)
- Modifying the physical environment (e.g. the provision of adaptive equipment, assistive technology or home modifications)
- Changing the social environment (e.g. training caregivers so that they can support someone more successfully)

In the example for Diana (in Chapter 11), we could suggest the following compensatory strategies:

- Encouraging Diana to use a computer, tablet or smartphone to keep her notes in order and to increase the displayed font size for her questions
- Using a recording device for interviews so Diana can concentrate on asking the questions and developing a relationship with the interviewee, rather than writing notes

Both these examples relate to the introduction of equipment, but this is not the only way we have to compensate for performance issues. If you think about your activity analysis (see Chapter 4) and are clear about the activity demands, you can identify aspects of the activity which could be changed. Figure 12.3 offers further examples of compensatory approaches related to individuals, groups and communities.

Compensatory approaches can be used with almost anyone, and can produce changes in a short space of time. Compensatory approaches can therefore be a good option if:

- You have limited time.
- Someone wants to achieve a goal quickly.
- Motivation is a barrier.
- Development of skills or body functions is too challenging.

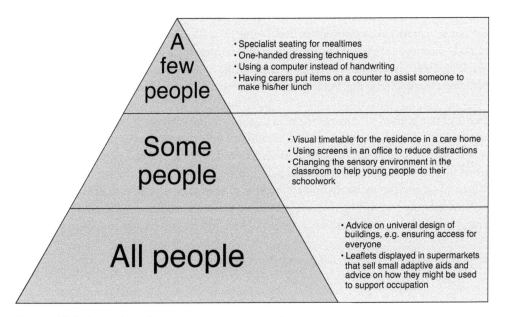

Figure 12.3 Examples of compensatory approaches

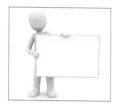

EDUCATOR EXAMPLES HERE:
COMPENSATORY INTERVENTION APPROACHES

– Provide additional resources or examples of compensatory intervention approaches relevant to the placement setting and clients.

SELECT A MODEL FOR EDUCATION AND TEACHING: PLAN AND IMPLEMENT EDUCATIONAL PROGRAMS FOR GROUPS FOCUSED ON PERFORMANCE OF DAILY LIFE TASKS

The focus of this intervention approach is to *educate*. Although all intervention approaches outlined in this model involve education, this approach focuses on educating groups of people about occupational performance, rather than focusing on a specific individual. For example, you might run a workshop for parents to support their child's transition between primary and secondary school.

The OTIPM reminds us to focus education sessions around our area of expertise: occupation. Do not be tempted to run workshops based solely on a diagnosis (e.g. cerebral palsy, autism) or body functions (e.g. motor, sensory). Instead, educate people on the potential impact of a diagnosis on occupational performance. Labelling the group based on occupational need (e.g. cooking, independent living, homework) will reinforce the focus of occupational therapy.

In the example given for Diana, one of her issues was the early morning starts. This may also be difficult for other students with disabilities in her journalism course. A suggestion might be to help her university lecturers understand the occupational needs of people with physical disabilities (including cerebral palsy) through offering a workshop. The intention here is to change the social environment (the staff members) so that they are more accommodating and willing to make reasonable adjustments. Figure 12.4 offers further examples of educational approaches related to individuals, groups and communities.

Educational approaches can be a good option when:

– There are similar concerns for a group of people which could be addressed effectively through training.
– There is value in promoting of the relationship of occupation to health and well-being to populations.

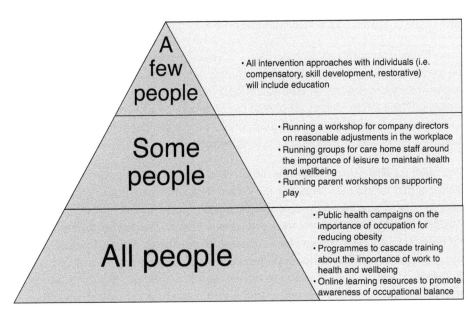

Figure 12.4 Examples of educational approaches

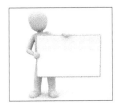

EDUCATOR EXAMPLES HERE:
EDUCATION-BASED INTERVENTION APPROACHES

....

- Provide additional resources or examples of education-based intervention approaches relevant to the placement setting and clients.

SELECT A MODEL FOR OCCUPATIONAL SKILLS TRAINING (ACQUISITIONAL MODEL): PLAN AND IMPLEMENT ACQUISITIONAL OCCUPATION TO RE-ACQUIRE OR DEVELOP OCCUPATIONAL SKILL

The intention of this intervention approach is to *develop occupational skills* (e.g. restore, develop, enhance or prevent loss of skills). Gaining or acquiring occupational skills could be through:

- Opportunities to practice performing meaningful and purposeful activities
- Grading activities so that the person can gradually develop skills
- Using a coaching approach to enable the development of clients' own problem-solving skills

In the example of Diana, skill development was the focus for two interventions:

- Using a coaching approach to help Diana develop an interview routine and the associated skills, then practicing the routine with role play and graded opportunities to develop the skills to conduct 'real' interviews
- Enabling Diana to develop strategies to become familiar with interview questions, such as having time to go through them prior to the interview, developing a bank of questions to draw from, writing her own questions etc.

The intention for *skill development* is for the client to develop skills required for occupational performance (i.e. enabling the person to learn to carry out activities, steps and actions – see Chapter 4 and your activity analysis). An example could be learning to tie your shoe laces by practicing the steps and using a rhyme to remember the sequence. This is likely to take longer and involve more effort to develop than compensatory interventions. For some people, however, development of skills is their priority (i.e. a child may want to tie his/her shoe laces to be like the other children). Skills may also be transferable to other contexts, depending on the person and how the skills are taught.

Compensatory and skill development approaches can appear similar. Again, what is important is your *intention* for the intervention. For example, if a person is having trouble finding items in a kitchen, we might put labels on the cupboards. If your intention is to leave the labels on the cupboard doors permanently, then this would be a compensatory approach. If, however, your intention is to help the person learn where things are located and gradually remove the labels as they develop skills, then it is a skill development (acquisitional) approach. Further examples are shown in Figure 12.5.

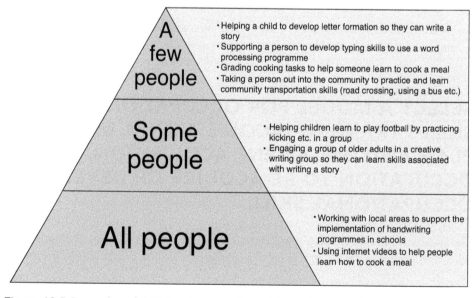

Figure 12.5 Examples of skill development (acquisitional) approaches

Acquisitional approaches can be a good option when:

- The person wants to change his/her skills in a valued occupation
- There is sufficient time to develop skills and incorporate them into daily life
- The person has the capacity and motivation to develop his/her skills

EDUCATOR EXAMPLES HERE:
SKILLS-BASED INTERVENTION APPROACHES

- Provide additional resources or examples of skills-based intervention approaches relevant to the placement setting and clients.

SELECT A MODEL FOR ENHANCEMENT OF PERSON FACTORS AND BODY FUNCTIONS (RESTORATIVE MODEL): PLAN AND IMPLEMENT RESTORATIVE OCCUPATION TO RESTORE OR DEVELOP PERSON FACTORS AND BODY FUNCTIONS

When the goal is to *restore* person factors or body functions, changes are made (through meaningful and purposeful activity) to develop or restore underlying body function or person factor components required for engaging in occupations, such as range of movement, motivation, mood, balance, fitness etc. The key here is that the activity used must be meaningful to the person, such as horse riding to develop core stability, working out at the gym to improve muscle strength, going to a social group to develop self-confidence, meditating to manage pain levels etc. Figure 12.6 outlines individual, group and community interventions based on a restorative approach.

In this approach, you reason that the development of these foundational abilities will likely result in increased occupational performance. It is important that you carefully monitor any impact on occupational performance as our occupational therapy theory and evidence suggests a more complex interplay of the person, environment and occupation

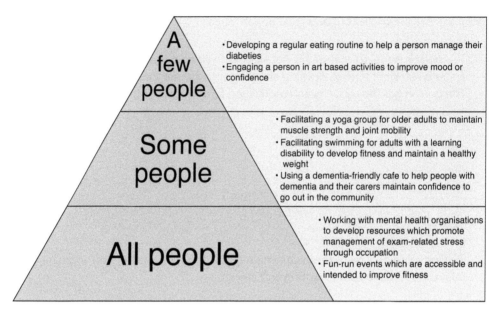

Figure 12.6 Examples of body-function and body-structure development approaches

which impacts on performance, rather than isolating individual body functions (e.g. Green and Payne, 2018). As Humphry (2002, p. 172) explains:

> Intervention models that explain acquisition of skills in daily activities in terms of changing a performance component, such as sensory integration or fine motor abilities, are of concern because evidence suggests that cognition, motor, sensory systems and emotion develop and operate simultaneously, so meaningful separation is questionable (Diamond, 2000; Magnusson, 2000; Thelen, 1995).

> Furthermore, suggesting internal change as the causal factor underlying development of occupation is not consistent with the conceptualization of occupation as emerging from person–environment interactions (Law et al., 2001).

The examples provided in Figure 12.6 emphasise the importance of engaging in meaningful occupation with a focus on developing, maintaining or restoring a body function. This contrasts with repetitive exercises or tasks which attempt to isolate an individual body function (e.g. stacking cones to improve shoulder mobility or placing pegs in a peg board to improve pincer grasp). These are not recommended because they are not meaningful occupations.

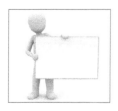

EDUCATOR EXAMPLES HERE:
RESTORATIVE INTERVENTION APPROACHES

....

– Provide additional resources or examples of restorative intervention approaches (if appropriate) relevant to the placement setting and clients.

MAKE A CHOICE OF APPROACH: USE YOUR PROFESSIONAL REASONING TO LINK YOUR ASSESSMENT FINDINGS TO YOUR INTERVENTIONS

In Chapter 11 you created a list of possible reasons for a client's challenges with occupational performance. You may have noticed that as you explain why you think the issues occurred, intervention ideas can become apparent.

In the example of Diana, a cluster was created from the occupational performance analysis about *initiates, continues, heeds* and *terminates*. The cluster was described as:

> Diana paused frequently during the task. For example, Diana hesitated before sitting down, paused before she retrieved her paper, notebook and pen and paused between asking questions. Diana also paused in the middle of asking questions and then wrote something and returned to asking the question. Diana stopped the interview before all the questions were asked and the supervisor took over the interview.

The possible reasons suggested for these challenges are described in Table 12.1. Each of these reasons would lead to a different intervention idea (as illustrated in the table).

It might be that a combination of factors contributed to the performance. Thus, you could try more than one strategy, either at the same time or one after another. You can then see which is most successful or most acceptable to those involved. Working in partnership with the client and significant others can help manage expectations about intervention outcomes and support people to remain motivated to try something else if the first thing does not work.

Think about how much the person and family can manage at one time. A balance of intervention approaches may be appropriate as strategies which involve skill development or enhancement of person factors/body functions are likely to take longer, while compensation and education could be effective while being less intensive and time consuming. For example, in Table 12.1, Diana wished to use her energy to develop skills in asking questions and conducting an interview. She decided that compensating for note writing (using a recording device) was acceptable as it enabled her to focus on her interpersonal skills.

It is also common for people to think of their own intervention ideas. If you spoke to Diana about your observations and possible reasons for the performance challenges, she may think of her own ways to change what is happening. This should be encouraged as it means Diana is taking ownership of the strategies (which is exactly what you want as you won't be there forever). Often people also come up with things you never thought of as they have a better understanding of their situation than you do. You don't need to have all the answers.

Table 12.1 Possible reasons for occupational performance challenges linked with intervention ideas

Possible reasons	Intervention ideas
Diana paused frequently as she was not familiar with the process of interviewing a person so she needed to think about each step every time.	Use a coaching approach to help Diana develop an interview routine. Practice the routine with role play and graded opportunities to conduct 'real' interviews. *(therapist intention: skill development)*
Diana was unfamiliar with the questions.	Support Diana to develop strategies to become familiar with interview questions such as having time to go through them prior to the interview, developing a bank of questions to draw from, writing her own questions etc. *(therapist intention: skill development)*
The notes were written in small font with lots of distracting notes.	Encourage Diana to use a computer, tablet or phone to record her questions. This will enable her to increase the font size and keep notes in order. *(therapist intention: compensatory)*
Due to her cerebral palsy, Diana wrote notes slowly.	Try using a recording device for interviews so Diana can concentrate on asking the questions and developing a relationship with the interviewee rather than writing notes. *(therapist intention: compensatory)*
Diana was fatigued due to the early morning start.	Try to schedule the interview for later in the morning or afternoon. *(therapist intention: compensatory)* In conjunction with Diana, run a workshop for Diana's lecturers about the potential impact of cerebral palsy on university work and reasonable adjustments. *(therapist intention: education)*

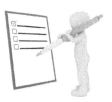

ACTIVITY

1   Using your own clusters and possible reasons lists from Chapter 11, write down some ideas about interventions which you think might address the performance challenges.
2   Discuss your ideas with your educator and peer in supervision.

CONSIDER WHAT ELSE CAN IMPACT ON INTERVENTION

There will be many factors involved in making reasoned decisions about which intervention approach to take. Your understanding of how people change; the interaction between the person, environment and occupation; and the purpose of an intervention contributes to the development of successful strategies. For example, you have knowledge of:

- The significance of the problems you identified during assessment
- What you realistically think can be achieved in the time you have with the client
- The person's goals and what approach he/she would be most comfortable with
- His/her person factors such as his/her level of motivation, internalised routines and self confidence
- His/her diagnosis and prognosis (e.g. does he/she have a deteriorating condition or condition/abilities that are unlikely to change?)
- The environment that he/she will perform in, whether you can adapt it and the amount of support that is available
- The person's financial situation
- The evidence-base for an approach

Change will need to be introduced at a pace which is acceptable to those involved. Perhaps begin with a minor change which is likely to have an immediate impact (such as adapting something in the environment or giving the person a piece of equipment). This will demonstrate the effectiveness of intervention and may help motivate staff members and clients for larger changes.

LOOK FOR INTERVENTION INSPIRATION OUTSIDE OF OCCUPATIONAL THERAPY

You may also draw upon other theories from outside of occupational therapy to support your reasoning and intervention approach. For example, in child and adolescent mental health you may draw on attachment theory (Bowlby, 1969; Crain, 2011) to consider how attachment problems might impact on the success of potential interventions. Sometimes you will be working in a team where theories or approaches are used by everyone in the team. For example, in an inpatient unit for adults with challenging behaviour, a cognitive-behavioural approach (Duncan, 2011; Wilson, 1978) may be routinely used.

These 'other' theories are sometimes referred to as *frames of reference* (see Chapter 3). Frames of reference can be useful to support conceptual models of occupational therapy practice (Duncan, 2011) and can help to guide us regarding *how* to do therapy

(Rodger, 2010). It is however important to recognise that when we use frames of reference as occupational therapists, we will implement them differently from other professionals, as we deliver them within our occupation-centred philosophy.

For example, an occupational therapist might work with someone who is anxious to develop skills in using public transport so that he/she can access their local leisure centre. The person may practice the journey and gradually reduce/grade the amount of support required as he/she develops skills. In this process, the occupational therapist may utilise cognitive-behavioural techniques (Duncan, 2011). This does not mean that the occupational therapist is practicing cognitive-behavioural therapy in the same way as a psychologist would; the occupational therapist can use techniques from that theory within the framework of occupational therapy (Boniface and Seymour, 2012).

REVIEW YOUR INTERVENTION IDEAS

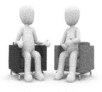

ACTIVITY

1   Revisit the intervention list you have created. Use these ideas as a basis for discussion with the client and significant others.
2   As with any intervention, it is important to consider the evidence-base. Look in the literature for evidence regarding an intervention and consider how this will influence your practice.
3   You may also like to revisit the Six Thinking Hats activity (Chapter 7) to help you to think about your intervention plan from different perspectives.

RISK ASSESSMENT

Prior to carrying out your intervention, consider if you need to complete a formal risk assessment. This will depend on the type of intervention you are proposing and it may be a requirement of the setting. Check with the local policy as there may be a standard risk assessment that you need to complete. Also, revisit Chapter 8 and the discussion about risk assessment.

CARRY OUT YOUR INTERVENTIONS

Uncertainty at this stage is a common feeling. Despite not knowing all the answers to your questions, you will need to try out your intervention ideas and learn from the results. If you have thought through your intervention carefully, discussed it with your educator and completed a risk assessment, you should feel confident to try out a strategy. *Remember that the strength of your interventions is also in the different perspectives you can offer for clients and setting staff.*

You are likely to find that when you begin trialling your strategies you will need to modify them based on the client's responses and the responses of others in the context; intervention is not just a one-off event. As you make changes, you will be constantly evaluating the difference in occupational performance and making further alterations. This is part of the cyclical occupational therapy process, indicated by the arrows in the OTIPM. *Follow the plan you have set, but be flexible.* If you feel that something should be changed when you are working with the client(s), then make those adaptations.

Remember to be as helpful as possible when you are trialling different strategies. For example, you may need to help re-arrange a room, or set up the lunch hall or make a visual timetable etc. Work closely with the setting staff members as they will carry this forward after you have finished your placement. Ensure the staff members have the necessary knowledge and materials to continue the interventions. You could create a 'how to' guide to help with this.

GAIN FEEDBACK ON YOUR PERFORMANCE

Following an intervention session, it will be important for you to reflect on your performance. You should ask for feedback from the client(s) and staff members you worked with. Your educator and/or peer may also like to observe you to provide specific feedback. To help with this, Figure 12.7 is example of a peer feedback form which you may like to use.

ACTIVITY

1   Arrange for a peer to observe you doing something with client(s) in your placement.
2   Consider using these notes as the basis of a reflection. How might you include this to inform your learning objectives?

Student observed: _____

Peer observer: _____

Activity observed: _____

Date: _____

Preparation

Was there evidence of the student preparing for the session in terms of:

- The environmental set up?
- The tools and equipment?
- Understanding of the person or group's needs?
- Was consent gained?

Content

Was the activity appropriate to the intervention aim?

Was the activity age appropriate?

Was an appropriate length of time allocated for completion of the activities?

Delivery

Were the session's goals clearly explained to participants?

Were communication strategies used effectively throughout the session?

Did the student recognise the need for grading and adaption of activities within the session?

Was the session appropriately ended?

Participant feedback

(Capture participants' feedback; consider both verbal and non-verbal feedback offered)

Following the session, use these prompts to engage in a discussion with your peer:

1 What worked well, what was good about the session?
2 What did not work so well, what could be changed or amended to improve the session?
3 What could the student do more of to develop their skills?

Peer signature: _____   Date: _____

Figure 12.7 Peer feedback form

CHAPTER SUMMARY

This chapter offered explanations of the four types of interventions outlined in the OTIPM: compensatory, educational, skill development and restorative. Example of using these intervention approaches with individuals, groups and communities were discussed. We described how you could include frames of reference within an occupation-centred perspective to add further detail to your intervention approach. Importantly, when you have reasoned thoroughly and considered any associated risks, you are encouraged to try out your intervention ideas. Through carrying out a plan and reflecting on the outcome and your own performance (with support from your educator and peer, if available), you can begin to judge the effectiveness of your involvement.

REFERENCES

Boniface G, Seymour A, eds (2012) *Using occupational therapy theory in practice*. Oxford, UK: Wiley-Blackwell.

Bowlby J (1969) *Attachment. Attachment and loss: Volume 1. Loss*. New York: Basic Books.

Case-Smith J, Arbesman M (2008) 'Evidence-based review of interventions for autism used in or of relevance to occupational therapy'. *American Journal of Occupational Therapy, 62*(4), 416–429.

Crain W (2011) *Theories of development: Concepts and applications*. 6th edn. Abingdon, Oxon: Routledge.

Dancza KM (2015) *Structure and uncertainty: The 'just right' balance for occupational therapy student learning on role-emerging placements in schools*. Doctor of Philosophy, The University of Queensland, Queensland, Australia.

Dancza KM, Missiuna C, Pollock N (2017) 'Occupation-centred practice: When the classroom or the school is your client'. In: S Rodger, A Kennedy-Behr, eds, *Occupation-centred practice with children: A practical guide for occupational therapists*. 2nd edn. West Sussex, UK: Wiley-Blackwell, pp. 257–287.

Diamond A (2000) 'Close interrelation of motor development and cognitive development and of the cerebellum and prefrontal cortex'. *Child Development, 71*, 44–56.

Duncan EAS, ed (2011) *Foundations for practice in occupational therapy*. 5th edn. Edinburgh, UK: Churchill Livingstone Elsevier.

Fisher AG (2009) *Occupational therapy intervention process model: A model for planning and implementing top-down, client centred, and occupation-based interventions*. Fort Collins, CO: Three Star Press.

Green D, Payne S (2018) 'Understanding organisational ability and self-regulation in children with Developmental Coordination Disorder'. Current Developmental Disorders Reports, Available https://doi.org/10.1007/s40474-018-0129-2 Accessed 28/01/18.

Humphry R (2002) 'Young children's occupations: Explicating the dynamics of developmental processes'. *American Journal of Occupational Therapy, 56*(2), 171–179.

Law M, Missiuna C, Pollock N, Stewart D (2001) 'Foundations for occupational therapy practice with children'. In: J Case-Smith, ed, *Occupational therapy for children*. 4th edn. St Louis, MO: Mosby, pp. 39–70.

Magnusson D (2000) 'The individual as the organizing principle'. In: LR Bergman, RB Cairns, L Nilsson, L Nystedt, eds, *Developmental science and the holistic approach*. Mahwah, NJ: Erlbaum, pp. 33–47.

Missiuna C, Pollock N, Levac DE, Campbell WN, Sahagian SD, Bennett SM, Hecimovich CA, Gaines BR, Cairney J and Russell DJ (2012) 'Partnering for change: An innovative school-based occupational therapy service delivery model for children with developmental coordination disorder'. *Canadian Journal of Occupational Therapy, 79*(1), 41–50.

Rodger S, ed (2010) *Occupation centred practice with children: A practical guide for Occupational Therapists*. West Sussex: Wiley-Blackwell.

Thelen E (1995) 'Motor development: A new synthesis'. *American Psychologist, 50*(2), 79–95.

Wilson GT (1978) 'Cognitive behavior therapy: Paradigm shift or passing phase?'. In: JP Foreyt, DP Rathjen, eds, *Cognitive behavioural therapy: Research and application*. New York: Springer, pp. 7–32.

World Health Organisation (2015–last update) *School health and youth health promotion*. [Homepage of World Health Organisation], [Online]. Available: www.who.int/school_youth_health/en/ [April 24, 2017].

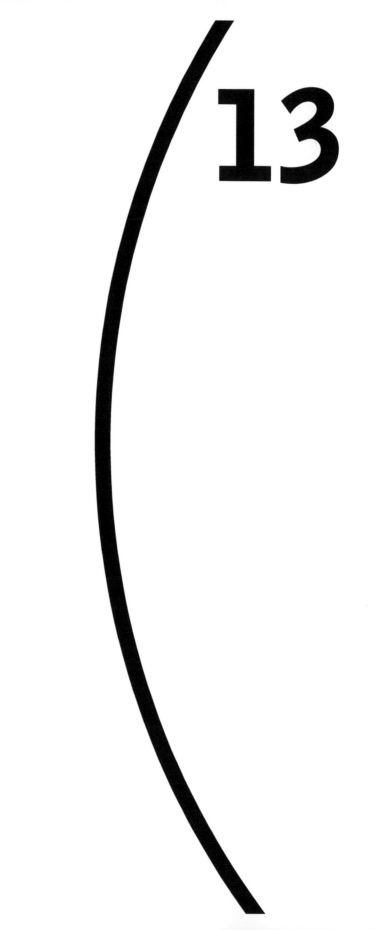

13

CHAPTER 13
RE-EVALUATION FOR ENHANCED AND SATISFYING OCCUPATIONAL PERFORMANCE

Monica Moran and Karina Dancza

INTENDED CHAPTER OUTCOMES

By the end of this chapter, readers will have an overview of:

- Different facets of evaluation, including client(s) changes in occupational performance, client(s) satisfaction with the changes, and the effectiveness and efficiency of the therapy process
- The bigger picture of how your contribution is evaluated at a service level
- Your responsibilities in terms of reporting requirements, hand-over and recommendations to ensure that service is seamlessly continued (or concluded)
- Evaluation of your learning goals (students) and supervision style (educators) and consideration of learning goals for the future

STAGE IN THE OTIPM

This chapter presents the re-evaluation phase within the Occupational Therapy Intervention Process Model (OTIPM; Fisher, 2009; see Figure 13.1). It is important to bear in mind that the OTIPM includes a large feedback loop, so while we may often think that re-evaluation occurs towards the end of the therapeutic process, it can occur at any time and feed back into the assessment and goal-setting phases.

INTRODUCTION

This concluding chapter in Part II introduces strategies for the re-evaluation of your service with clients. This will include how we link the re-evaluation process with the baseline assessment information (Chapter 6). We will also explore strategies for updating and finalising your reports and recommendations. This will assist in a smooth continuation or conclusion of service as you prepare for ending your placement.

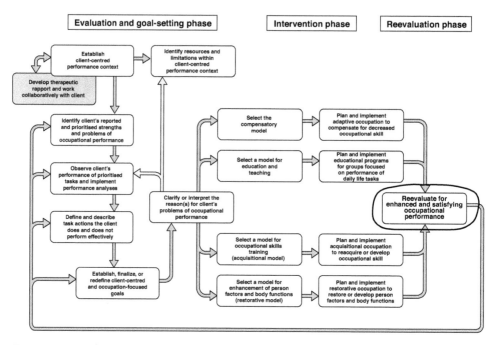

Figure 13.1 Schematic representation of the steps in the OTIPM – Re-evaluation phase

Adapted from Fisher (2009). Available: www.innovativeotsolutions.com/content/wp-content/uploads/2014/01/English-OTIPM-handout.pdf. Reprinted with permission.

It is likely that you will be evaluating the service you provided with an individual or group of clients. In addition to this, thinking about how your work contributes to overall service provision is important preparation for your work when you graduate.

The closing section of this chapter contains information on ways to evaluate your learning using a range of strategies including self-evaluation, peer evaluation and educator evaluation.

WHAT IS RE-EVALUATION?

When you have implemented your intervention and you are coming to the end of your placement, you will need to ensure you have *time to re-evaluate the priority area(s)* you focused on. There are many ways in which you can do this. Before we explore the detail of re-evaluation, it is useful to think about what we mean when we talk about 'goals', 'outcomes' and 'evaluations'. The English Oxford Living Dictionary (https://en.oxforddictionaries.com/) provides the following definitions.

- **Goals**: "the object of a person's ambition or effort; an aim or desired result"
- **Outcomes**: "the way a thing turns out; a consequence"
- **Evaluations**: "the making of a judgement about the amount, number, or value of something"

We described *goals* in Chapter 10 and discussed how these are a source of motivation for clients. Goals were then refined so we could focus our interventions and determine how to measure success. *Outcomes* are the way the goal turned out following our intervention. Taking that one step further, an *outcome evaluation* can be thought of as making a judgement about the effectiveness or value of these outcomes.

For example, if the goal was to cook a meal for the family and the outcome was that a meal was cooked, an outcome evaluation may consider how frequently this cooking happens, the range of meals cooked, the quality and complexity of the meals, and how satisfied the client is with his/her cooking.

You may also consider how effective and efficient the service was that you provided. One part of this evaluation is the client's opinion of your performance. This will have a direct influence on his/her commitment to collaborating with you and continuing with the strategies or approach after you finish your placement. Other aspects of your performance to consider are:

- How you used evidence to inform your approach with clients
- The strategies you used to challenge your assumptions as you reasoned and planned your interventions (e.g. discussions with more experienced colleagues)
- How you allocated your time and if there was sufficient time for changes to be seen in occupational performance

CREATING A RE-EVALUATION PLAN

How you measure the success (or not) of your intervention depends on the questions you want to answer. For example:

- Has the intervention changed the occupational performance of clients? If so, how?
- Have clients achieved the occupational goal they jointly developed with me?
- Did the clients receive the best (most evidence based) intervention from me?
- Are the clients satisfied with the service I have provided?
- Did the clients receive services from me in a timely way?
- Can the clients continue to work on their goals?
- Are my recommendations for follow-up timely and appropriate?

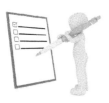

ACTIVITY

1   Generate a list of the evaluation questions you would like to answer about the work you have completed.
2   From the list you generated, who are you seeking the opinions of? Consider the following:
    –   Your own opinion and professional judgement
    –   The opinions and professional judgements of your educator and other team members
    –   The opinions and experiences of clients

We call this approach to re-evaluation a 'pluralistic approach' (Hart, 1999). This approach acknowledges that there is a range of different stakeholders and evaluation tools you can use in your practice.

STRATEGIES AND TOOLS FOR RE-EVALUATION

Your re-evaluation plan and tools will be informed by the questions you wish to answer and the information you gathered earlier in the occupational therapy process. Consider:

–   Reviewing the goals set with clients (see Chapter 10)
–   Re-interviewing clients
–   Re-interviewing the setting staff members (e.g. what has changed in the practice setting? Are people doing things differently?)
–   Reflecting on whether your presence or role in the organisation has changed the way team members see occupational therapy
–   Observing the priority area(s) and completing another occupational performance analysis to compare with your original
–   Re-photographing the environment

Discuss with your educator what evaluation tools are available at your placement location to help you answer these questions. Tools to help you in the re-evaluation phase are numerous and evolving.

Some evaluation tools can support your occupational therapy process. For example, *The Canadian Occupational Performance Measure* (COPM; Law, Baptiste, Carswell, McColl,

Polatajko and Pollock, 2014) can help with goal setting; *The Pediatric Evaluation of Disability Inventory* (PEDI; Haley, Coster, Ludlow, Haltiwanger and Andrellos, 1992) can help your initial interview to find out about a range of life areas where clients may need your involvement. With these types of tools, you can compare the original scores with those you collect following your intervention.

Other tools can appear to have a more distant focus, but are often used for evaluating at a service or population level or where there are multiple professional groups involved. Examples of these tools include:

- *Therapy Outcome Measures* (TOMS; Enderby and John, 2015)
- *Australian Therapy Outcomes Measures* (AUSTOMS; Unsworth, 2014)
- *EQ-5D* (The EuroQol Group, 1990)
- *Health of the Nation Outcome Scales* (HoNOS; Wing, Curtis and Beevor, 1996)

As highlighted in Chapter 7, there may be challenges in attempting to use tools which have been developed in a different country or setting from where you are currently working. Discuss with your educator the suitability of any tool you plan on using in your re-evaluation.

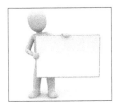

EDUCATOR EXAMPLES HERE:
EVALUATION TOOLS

- Where possible, provide examples of evaluation tools which the student(s) may come across in your setting.
- Discuss with the student(s) how you would like them to be used during the placement.

SUMMATIVE VERSUS FORMATIVE RE-EVALUATION

When we think about re-evaluation, we often think of a process that occurs towards the end of the therapy cycle. However, the reality is slightly more fluid. You may be familiar with the terms 'formative' and 'summative' from your university programs. *Formative* refers to an ongoing evaluation throughout the therapeutic process, while *summative* refers to a final evaluation at the end of the therapeutic process.

Consider how you conduct brief re-evaluations with your clients every time you see them. You may use observation, informal interview and brief assessment to answer questions about your client's experience and changes in their occupational performance. You probably use this *formative* information to carefully modify your interventions. Evaluation as a *formative* activity ensures that you are constantly modifying your interventions in response to the changing needs and capabilities of your clients.

Summative re-evaluations completed at a defined time point with your client provide a more definite set of data that you can use to answer questions about client outcomes, efficacy of therapy, client satisfaction etc. This vital information offers you indications of the next steps for your client and will feed into your recommendations for further intervention, follow up or discharge. Summative evaluation is also likely to be important to feed into wider service level evaluations.

ACTIVITY
....

Prepare the following questions for discussion with your educator:

– What have you been *formatively* re-evaluating during the occupational therapy process?
– What is your plan for your *summative* re-evaluation?
– What re-evaluation tools or methods will you use?
– Why will you use these tools or methods?
– How will you document the results of your re-evaluations?

SERVICE EVALUATION – WHAT'S IT GOT TO DO WITH ME?

All services, whether they are occupational therapy–specific or inter-professional, are funded by commissioning or funding organisations. If you are completing your placement with a private practitioner, it is very clear who is paying for the services you provide. If you are placed in a public health service (e.g. public hospital) it may be less clear who is paying for services. If you are in a non-government organisation (NGO), services may be linked to short-term funded contracts. In each of these situations the funders (payers) will have expectations that service providers can evidence the value of the services that they are providing. This may include information about client outcomes and efficiency of service delivery including cost effectiveness, client satisfaction, timeliness of service delivery, staff skill mix and many other criteria. As a student, your involvement contributes to the overall performance of the service.

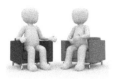

ACTIVITY
....

1   Ask your educator about the service/program re-evaluation activities that must be completed in your placement location.
2   List how your activities contribute to these program evaluation activities.

FINALISING YOUR REPORT

You will need to finalise your involvement with the intervention(s) and ensure that plans are in place for you to hand these over to the client(s) and relevant staff members when you leave. Go back to the report you wrote and add in the specific intervention information and the feedback from your re-evaluation (see Chapter 9 for examples). You may also need to add in future recommendations if there are aspects which could be acted on after you finish your placement. The service setting may also like a summary report of your involvement in each of your project areas. You will need to ensure that all your notes and reports are counter-signed by your educator (if required) and are securely filed in line with the documentation management protocols of the setting.

FINALISING YOUR LEARNING DOCUMENTS

Prior to the end of your placement, ensure that your placement paperwork is updated and your learning objectives/outcomes reflect any new insights you have gained. One of your final tasks may be looking back on earlier reflections and seeing how you have progressed during the placement.

Whilst your intervention suggestions will hopefully have made a positive impact on the clients' occupations, it is also likely that you have supported the setting staff members through offering a unique perspective. Do not under-estimate the value of reframing perspectives of clients and those involved with the clients, as it is possible that this will have a lasting impact.

When you are re-evaluating your own learning, consider gathering information from a variety of sources such as:

−   Self-evaluation
−   Peer evaluation
−   Educator evaluation
−   Client evaluation

There is a range of tools which can support you gathering this information. Chapter 12 gave an example of a peer feedback form which you could use. The *individual Teamwork Observation and Feedback Tool* (iToFT; Thistlethwaite et al., 2016) is another freely available tool for student self and peer evaluation when you are working as part of an inter-professional team. It can be downloaded from the Australian Awards for University Teaching website (www.olt.gov.au/project-work-based-assessment-teamwork-interprofessional-approach-2012). It provides qualitative feedback on your performance while you are learning and allows you to use the feedback to improve your performance.

RE-EVALUATION IDEAS FOR EDUCATORS

As part of your re-evaluation of your supervision, consider:

1   How have these students changed your practice?
2   Through working with these students, have you been introduced to innovative ways of thinking about your practice or looked at different ways to practice?
3   How will you feedback to the students the ways in which they have changed your thinking?
4   How have your skills as a supervisor developed or evolved through working with these students?
5   What supervisory skills would you like to develop further and how might you make this happen?

CHAPTER SUMMARY

This chapter presented the last step in your occupational therapy process: you re-evaluated the occupational performance of the client, his/her satisfaction and the efficacy of your involvement. We considered how you could design and implement an evaluation plan in relation to the clients, along with how you would evaluate your own learning as a student or educator.

CONGRATULATIONS!

You have come to the end of your placement, hopefully with a better understanding of what it is to be an occupational therapist and how important and helpful it is to use theory to guide your practice. Take time to reflect on the challenges you have experienced and the successes you have achieved. This is just the beginning of your learning journey which will continue throughout your career as an occupational therapist. *Well done!*

REFERENCES

Enderby P, John A, eds (2015) *Therapy outcome measures for rehabilitation professionals.* 3rd edn. Guildford: J & R Press Ltd.

EuroQol Group (1990) 'EuroQol – A new facility for the measurement of health-related quality of life'. *Health Policy, 16*(3), 199–208.

Fisher AG (2009) *Occupational Therapy intervention process model: A model for planning and implementing top-down, client centred, and occupation-based interventions.* Fort Collins, CO: Three Star Press.

Haley SM, Coster WJ, Ludlow LH, Haltiwanger JT, Andrellos PA (1992) *Pediatric Evaluation of disability inventory: Development, standardization and administration manual.* Boston, MA: Trustees of Boston University.

Hart E (1999) 'The use of pluralistic evaluation to explore people's experiences of stroke services in the community'. *Health & Social Care in the Community, 7*, 248–256.

Law M, Baptiste S, Carswell A, McColl MA, Polatajko H, Pollock N (2014) *Canadian Occupational Performance Measure (COPM).* 5th edn. Ottawa, ON: Canadian Association of Occupational Therapists.

Oxford (2017–last update) *English Oxford living dictionary.* Available: https://en.oxforddictionaries.com/ [April 20, 2017].

Thistlethwaite J, Dallest K, Moran M, Dunston R, Roberts C, Eley D . . . Fyfe S (2016) 'Introducing the individual Teamwork Observation and Feedback Tool (iTOFT): Development and description of a new interprofessional teamwork measure'. *Journal of Interprofessional Care, 30*, 526–528.

Unsworth C (2014) *Australian Therapy Outcomes Measures (AUSTOMS).* Available: https://austoms.com [July 10, 2017].

Wing JK, Curtis RH, Beevor AS (1996) *HoNOS: Health of the Nation Outcome Scales: Report on Research and Development July 1993–December 1995.* London: Royal College of Psychiatrists.

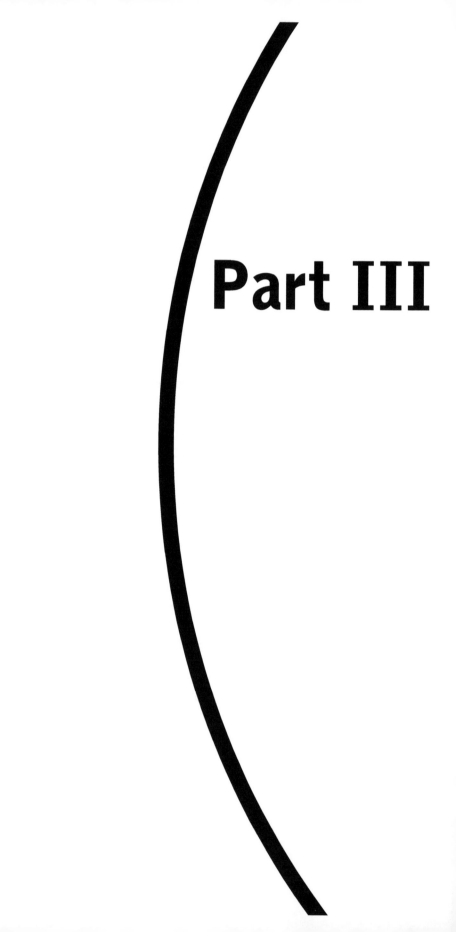

Part III

ADVICE FOR EDUCATORS AND CASE STUDIES

OVERVIEW

Part III is primarily written with educators in mind, although as described by Dr. Hooper in her foreword to this book, students may also appreciate the insights offered into the learning processes and use of occupation-centred principles in different service settings.

This section opens with Chapter 14, which provides an overview of educational theory and its relevance to occupational therapy practice learning. The chapter also introduces educators to the Professional Learning through Useful Support (PLUS) Framework, which highlights critical areas for practice learning and offers recommendations for educators in how to support future practitioners to enact occupation-centred principles.

Throughout this book we have prompted educators to offer students relevant contextualisation of materials to local practice learning settings to maximise the book's potential. This is consistent with the educational ideas presented in Chapter 14.

The final two chapters in Part III are intended to support this contextualisation and comprise six case study examples of how this book (in draft form) has been used by educators and students in role-emerging and role-established placements in Australia, the United Kingdom and Canada. They highlight some of the successes and challenges we as educators have experienced, along with some of our learning.

The authors of these case studies openly shared their personal reflections, concerns and strategies as they supported student practice learning. These honest accounts do not attempt to 'sugar coat' the real struggles they experienced. Whilst attempts have been made to anonymise these experiences, it is impossible to de-identify all aspects. We therefore respectfully ask the reader to be mindful of the privilege it is to have these reflections shared. It is hoped that through doing this, you may know you are not alone if you have some similar experiences.

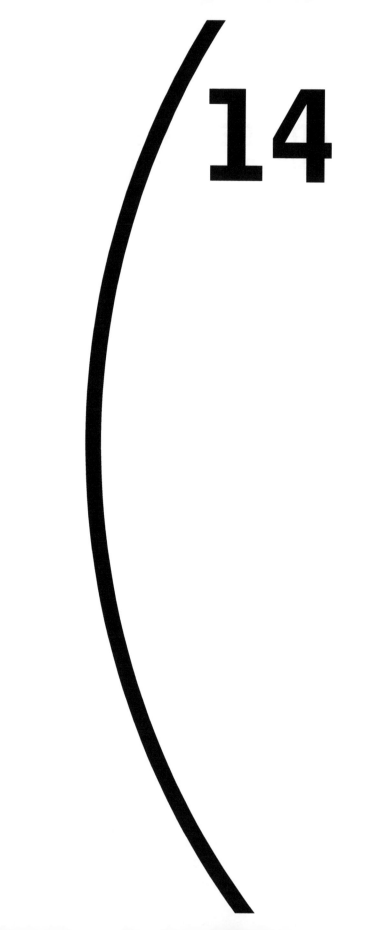

14

CHAPTER 14
EDUCATION PRINCIPLES FOR LEARNING

Karina Dancza, Anita Volkert and Monica Moran

INTENDED CHAPTER OUTCOMES

By the end of this chapter, readers will have an overview of:

- The relationship between student education experiences and the development of professional identity
- Contemporary educational theories informing occupational therapy education
- The Professional Learning through Useful Support (PLUS) Framework, which aids educators to consolidate and develop in their supervisory role

INTRODUCTION

This book is concerned with the development of occupation-centred practice (as presented in Chapters 2–4), in the context of practice learning. Practice learning is fundamental to the development of professional identity in students. In this chapter, we will examine the development of professional identity as it evolves during practice learning experiences. We will then explore some key learning theories that we have found helpful in understanding practice learning. Finally, we describe the Professional Learning through Useful Support (PLUS) Framework (Dancza, 2015), which applies learning principles directly to practice learning. Each element of the PLUS Framework is described and its congruence with the wider practice and university context is explored.

The intention of this chapter is not to provide a comprehensive account of educational theory; rather it is to demonstrate how theory can link with real experiences so we can understand and develop enriched learning opportunities. This chapter and the PLUS Framework are aimed at supporting educators in scaffolding students' practice learning. Students may also find it interesting to consider their own learning processes from an educational theory perspective.

PROFESSIONAL IDENTITY

The development and consolidation of professional identity is a key feature of practice learning (Ashby, Adler and Herbert, 2016). The professional socialisation which occurs when students apply learning in authentic situations is a powerful influence on the development of students' professional identity (Sabari, 1985; Lindquist, Engardt, Garnham, Poland and Richardson, 2006). This means that students learn about the profession from placement experiences as much as, and perhaps more than, from their university education.

Molineux (2011) suggested that for occupational therapy students to develop their professional identity, occupation-centred practice must be the cornerstone of the curriculum. While this is obviously important, an occupation-centred focus at university may not be enough if it is not reinforced in practice (Towns and Ashby, 2014). Ideally, students need consistency between the major concepts they learn at university and what they observe as the role of the occupational therapist in placement.

The development of a strong and consistent professional identity can be a protective factor for students and professionals to remain resilient in uncertain working contexts (Ashby, Ryan, Gray and James, 2013). Professional identity is not, however, a static and tangible construct. It is not something which is obtained by students and then used as a 'protective shield' to ensure they undertake occupational therapy roles and are not drawn into other professional domains. Professional identity is dynamic and evolving (Dancza, 2015).

For example, in the study by Dancza (2015), at the beginning of a role-emerging placement students expressed some ideas about their role. It was, however, only through exploration of their ideas during placement and engagement with critical debates with their peer and educator, that they consolidated their professional identity. Clear, but flexible, guidance was required to enable students to apply occupation-centred theory to practice and support the development of their professional identity.

A metaphor which could be used to illustrate the dynamics of the guidance between the student and educator is of a person flying a kite. The educator and student are connected throughout the placement, much like a person (the educator) holding the kite (the student) by the string. The educator releases the string to allow the student freedom and flexibility to practice, or draws the student back if he/she is moving away from his/her core tasks. The connection via the string symbolises the explicit guidance between the educator and student that links and reinforces theory with practice. This constant adjustment occurs depending on the 'weather conditions' or practice and university contexts, which require careful handling during the placement (see Figure 14.1).

The way in which educators make these constant adjustments in their supervisory role is something which is often developed through experience. We can, however, also use educational theory to help us better understand the learning processes of students, so we can make these often-unconscious adjustments more explicit.

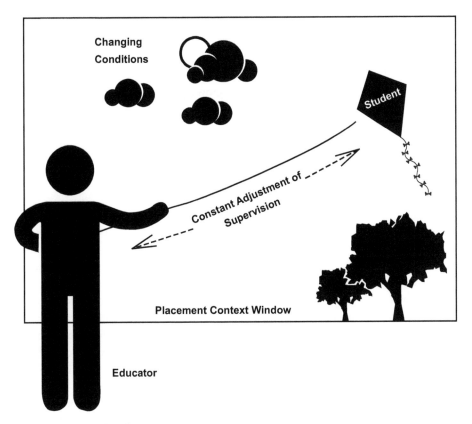

Figure 14.1 Metaphor for supervision

EDUCATIONAL THEORY APPLIED TO OCCUPATIONAL THERAPY EDUCATION

Occupational therapists are familiar with using theory to inform their practice with different client groups (as explored in Chapter 3). Less well developed is the overt use of educational theory to inform how we develop future occupational therapists (Hooper, King, Wood, Bilics and Gupta, 2013).

Occupational therapy as a profession is still engaged in articulating the processes we follow to create and foster a sense of professional identity in students, new graduates and experienced practitioners (Turner, 2011). We face several challenges and opportunities as we move forward in education, practice, leadership and research in the twenty-first century. These include changing health, social care and education policy contexts which have resulted in both a reduction in traditional roles for occupational therapists and an increase in emergent roles (Kronenberg, Pollard and Sakellariou, 2011). Practitioners engaging in these roles need a keen sense of professional self, an openness to working in entirely new multidisciplinary team constructs, resilience, and a clear grasp of occupation-centred practice and the accompanying professional reasoning.

The Royal College of Occupational Therapist's Career Development Framework in the United Kingdom (RCOT, 2017) emphasises the importance of occupation-centred practice within its four pillars of practice: Professional Practice, Facilitation of Learning, Leadership and Evidence, and Research and Development. Frameworks such as this offer guidance as we exploit future opportunities for growth in the profession.

With these opportunities comes new demands for the profession. For example, experienced practitioners who act as educators, supervisors and mentors will need to develop their own knowledge and skills to support the professionals of the future (Volkert, 2017). Understanding student learning using contemporary educational theories may be one way to support educators to meet this challenge.

The metaphor of learning as an experience leading to a state of personal or professional transformation has been formally described in several key theories and frameworks in the educational literature. Amongst the most influential is Transformational Learning Theory (Mezirow, 2000), however a range of other educational theories also reflect a transformative learning journey. These theories and frameworks have much to offer occupational therapy practice education as they broadly articulate a move away from task-orientated learning processes, to a more complex and nuanced experience involving a transformative change within the learner. Several key theories and frameworks are briefly described here. Please note that this is not an exhaustive nor a static list, but it does offer a starting point for reflection.

Transformative learning theory (Mezirow, 1997) provides a set of conditions to facilitate the learner to develop autonomous thinking, challenge the learner's pre-existing beliefs, create new meanings and help the learner to become self-reflective. From this perspective, as learners develop their understanding of concepts or practices they undergo a transformation which changes their sense of identity.

The threshold concepts framework (Fortune and Kennedy-Jones, 2014; Rodger and Turpin, 2011; Tanner, 2011) suggests that all disciplines have unique ways of knowing and practicing. Only when students have engaged and traversed a learning "threshold" (p. 4) will troublesome concepts or practices become clear (Cousin, 2006). Progression through these thresholds is transformative: not only are these concepts about integrating new information, but also about letting go of some previously held and prevailing beliefs. This is often an uncomfortable and emotional experience (Meyer and Land, 2005). Once students have moved through this learning threshold they are changed irreversibly and cannot go back to a previous way of thinking.

Another educational theory that incites transformation in the learner is *action learning theory* (Schon, 1983), which involves 'doing' in real situations. It is also often referred to as *authentic* or *experiential learning* and is the basis of practice learning. This style of learning is usually considered to involve action (doing), discussion (words), and a context in which the actions and discussions take place (Schon, 1983). Similarly, *experiential learning theory*

(Kolb, 1984) suggests that new knowledge is created through a process of engagement in a situation (the 'doing'), *reflection* on these experiences, and *interpreting* and *applying* new understandings to subsequent situations.

In summary, all these theories and frameworks can be seen to have somewhat similar components: deep engagement with an experience (the learning task), in an authentic setting, the challenging of existing attitudes or belief sets, critical self-reflection and discussion, and creation of new meanings. This set of conditions is seen to facilitate a transformation within the learner towards a new professional identity.

Practical examples of how to use educational theories to scaffold student practice learning to facilitate transformational learning experiences are presented through the PLUS Framework. This was developed as a tool for educators to help articulate the sticking points for students during practice learning, so that focused support can be provided. It is also intended to offer a way for educators to reflect on and enhance their own supervisory performance.

PLUS FRAMEWORK

The PLUS Framework (Figure 14.2) is an educational tool created to describe a set of guidance strategies used by skilled educators to support student practice learning, whilst acknowledging the critical influences of the practice and university contexts. The PLUS Framework offers a set of strategies for achieving ongoing adjustment or a 'just-right balance' between developing a clear structure and procedures for students to follow, and requiring students to make active decisions to facilitate their own independent learning and development of professional identity (Dancza, 2015).

The central construct of the PLUS Framework is student learning. This is surrounded by three Focal Points (sticking points) with key strategies that educators can use to facilitate student learning. Each Focal Point comprises several strategies which are not hierarchal in nature. Each of the strategies are required at various times and levels of intensity throughout the placement. The overarching strategies are:

1 Guide learning
2 Reflect on your own theory-to-practice links
3 Challenge perceptions

Surrounding these Focal Points are the practice and university contexts. Both aspects influence students and educators through the availability of resources, attitudes towards and expectations of the students, and the education and preparation of all stakeholders. The following sections offer a detailed exploration of each of these Focal Points and accompanying strategies.

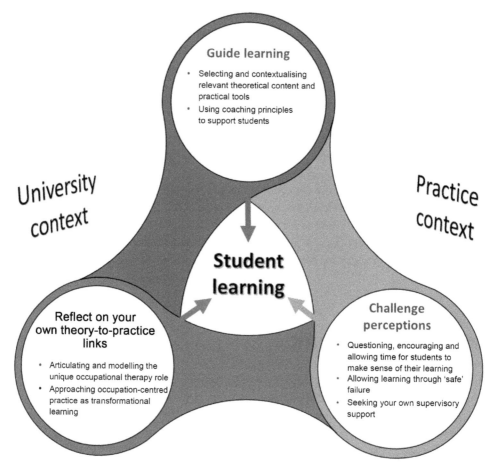

Figure 14.2 PLUS Framework
Adapted from Dancza (2015).

FOCAL POINT 1: GUIDE LEARNING

The overarching strategy in the first Focal Point is to *guide learning* of the students through:

1.1   Selecting and contextualising relevant theoretical content and practical tools
1.2   Using coaching principles to support students

FOCAL POINT 1.1: SELECTING AND CONTEXTUALISING
RELEVANT THEORETICAL CONTENT AND PRACTICAL TOOLS

Your focus as an educator is to choose and adapt relevant theories, models and tools so that students achieve the knowledge and skills required to practice as an occupational therapist. Curricular content is often guided by national or international professional bodies and regulatory authorities, such as the World Federation of Occupational

Therapists (WFOT, 2002), the Health and Care Professions Council (UK) (HCPC, 2013) and the Royal College of Occupational Therapists (UK) (RCOT, 2008). As an educator, you also make many choices about what to include in the curriculum, such as which models and frames of reference to teach, and importantly, how content is delivered (RCOT, 2008).

Whilst this selection and contextualisation of theories, models and tools in the curriculum helps students focus on relevant aspects of occupational therapy, it is often insufficient for their practice learning. It may be necessary for the educator to further select, filter and reframe theory to help students make sense of the plethora of options available to them (Dancza, 2015).

This concept of selecting, filtering and reframing theory and tools was used throughout Part II with the 'educator examples here' prompts (see Chapter 1 for more details). The suggested contextualisation was devised through the original research for this book (Dancza, Copley, Rodger and Moran, 2016). The Occupational Therapy Intervention Process Model (OTIPM; Fisher, 2009) and resources provide a mechanism for making the implicit and tacit knowledge of occupational therapy practice explicit – a key task in the process of supervision and mentoring (Morrison and Robertson, 2016).

FOCAL POINT 1.2: USING COACHING PRINCIPLES TO SUPPORT STUDENTS

Coaching has been used within occupational therapy primarily as a therapeutic tool with clients (Kessler and Graham, 2015), but has also received some attention within student education as an alternative approach to mentoring (Huggins, 2016). Coaching strategies include offering emotional support, providing information which is timely and specific for the situation and following a structured process (Graham, Rodger and Kennedy-Behr, 2017).

Emotional support is required during placement as transformative learning is frequently uncomfortable (Meyer and Land, 2003). Discomfort is a natural part of learning, particularly when a threshold concept (e.g. occupation-centred practice) is being mastered. Discomfort can be heightened when you challenge (question) students about their understanding of these concepts. Questioning assists students to develop critical reasoning. It is also important for students to develop strategies that lead to emotional resilience in their future workplaces. Being open with students about potential challenges, recognising when emotions are heightened, and providing time and discussion opportunities are all useful approaches for demonstrating emotional support.

Timely and specific information is required as students can become overwhelmed with uncertainty during placements. As an educator, you may have experienced times where students have not appreciated the relevance of practical skills, particularly if they were presented at university where they were not able to immediately apply them. *Situated learning theory* (Lave and Wenger, 1991) helps us to understand why this may be so.

To consolidate knowledge learnt in the university context it is important that placement opportunities allow for learning to be revisited and used within authentic or real situations. For example, students may learn about interviewing a person in relation to their occupational needs at university and role-play these skills with peers or others. It may only be when they are on placement that students see the need for interviewing and appreciate the importance of the techniques they have been exposed to. Timely and specific reinforcement of theory with students, directing them back to their university learning, providing opportunities to practice in real situations and critically reviewing these experiences are ways which can support student learning.

Timely information is also reflected in the structure of this book. Part II follows the student's placement timeline and the OTIPM (Fisher, 2009) process, so that guidance is graduated and presented at the appropriate time.

In addition, student and supervisor preparation for placement also needs to be timely. The two weeks prior to placement appear critical for preparation as students can see the immediate relevance for their work. Chapter 5 offers some key preparation strategies for students and educators.

A structured process such as the use of the OTIPM (Fisher, 2009), benefits both students and educators. It enables students to see the wider picture of their placement and establish exactly where they are within the process at any given point in time. This is consistent with novice practitioner's preference for following pre-determined routines (Unsworth, 2001) and reflects competency theory (Dreyfus and Dreyfus, 1986). You will, however, need to regularly direct students back to the process during supervision to help them continue to make links between theory and practice. This is illustrated in the case study Chapters 15 and 16.

FOCAL POINT 2: REFLECT ON YOUR OWN THEORY-TO-PRACTICE LINKS

The overarching strategy for the second Focal Point is for educators to *reflect on their own theory to practice links* by:

2.1   Articulating and modelling the unique occupational therapy role
2.2   Approaching occupation-centred practice as a piece of transformative learning

FOCAL POINT 2.1: ARTICULATING AND MODELLING THE UNIQUE OCCUPATIONAL THERAPY ROLE

Articulating and modelling the occupational therapy role may appear straightforward; but it often is not. It is not unusual for experienced occupational therapists to make decisions about their practice intuitively, which makes it difficult for students to follow their reasoning process.

Using theory to guide and explain reasoning makes intuitive decisions explicit. Some authors, however, have written of the hesitancy of occupational therapy practitioners to explain how they use theory to guide decision making (Du Toit and Wilkinson, 2011; Ikiugu, 2012). This is problematic for students as without an explicit focus on the use of theory, students can be drawn into 'assistant' or 'helper' roles as they copy the actions of a more experienced person without clear understanding of what they are doing and why (Wilding and Whiteford, 2007).

To make connections explicit for students, we need to clarify our own understanding of occupational therapy theory and how it guides our practice. This could be particularly challenging if we are also grappling with occupation-centred practice. Focusing on the occupational needs of the people, facilitating the supervision of students using a model such as the OTIPM (Fisher, 2009) and critically reflecting with other educators through peer support are all ways to address these challenges.

FOCAL POINT 2.2: APPROACHING OCCUPATION-CENTRED PRACTICE AS TRANSFORMATIVE LEARNING

Thinking about occupation-centred practice as requiring transformative learning, or more specifically *as a threshold concept* can be a useful way of understanding the emotional fluctuations and challenges students' experience (Rodger and Turpin, 2011; Tanner, 2011).

For example, you may see students understand the occupational needs of a client and develop ideas to support his/her occupational performance during a supervision session. Between supervision sessions students may move away from these ideas and be swayed by other practices or professionals (such as focusing on running established groups to improve confidence of clients or supporting the physiotherapist to implement an exercise programme through activity). A discussion of top-down, bottom-up and top-to-bottom up reasoning (as described in Chapter 2) may help students see these differing perspectives.

While this oscillation in understanding can be evident to educators, students often cannot independently recognise when this occurs and often inadvertently label their practice incorrectly. For example, during the initial weeks of placement students may use terms to describe their practice which they know are professionally important, such as being 'occupation-centred', 'person-centred' and 'holistic' in their views. When pressed by educators to explain, students often struggle to articulate exactly how these concepts relate to, and influence, the assessment and intervention processes they are proposing. Students may find that when pushed by educators to discuss their reasoning it can be forced or artificial in nature. From a threshold concept lens, this is referred to as 'mimicry', whereby the students tell educators what they want to hear, as opposed to really understanding the meaning underpinning the concept (Cousin, 2006). This was described by Fortune and Kennedy-Jones (2014) as illustrative of Meyer and Land's (2003) state of 'liminality'. This is where uncertainty is paramount until the learning threshold is crossed.

This period of uncertainty is known as liminal space. Students oscillate in this liminal space until they have an 'ah ha' moment where the concept is illuminated. From this point, there is no going back (irreversibility).

Support is critical whilst students navigate this liminal state in their understanding of occupation-centred practice (Cousin, 2006). Using the OTIPM (Fisher, 2009) and this book, accessing literature and peer support are often not enough. Students require strong encouragement and ongoing discussion about the reasons for the decisions they are making with their educator to challenge their understanding of occupation-centred practice and scaffold their learning (Chaiklin, 2003; Vygotsky, 1978). Supporting students to reflect on their practice and learning is also critical. Keeping a record of their thinking and reasoning (such as through a reflective journal) will mean students can use reflection to think about their ongoing actions, but it can also be used to look back on how their reasoning has developed.

This is especially important as, towards the latter stages of the placement when students experience the occupational therapy process and have some successes regarding their interventions, their understanding of occupation-centred practice often evolves to an extent that they can no longer recall the journey that they have been through. 'Forgetting' these challenges can mean that when students become educators themselves, they may experience their own frustrations at the fluctuations in learning of the next cohort of occupational therapy students! Looking back on their previous reflections can help them see how far their learning has developed.

For educators, understanding occupation-centred practice from a transformative learning and threshold concept perspective may offer some clarity as to these learning processes. It may also offer some reassurance that the educator's own understanding of occupation-centred practice could be evolving alongside the students and this may account for some of the discomfort they experience in their supervisory role. Whilst in liminal space, individuals need support from both peers who are in the same space and experienced mentors/supervisors who can scaffold and direct learning experiences and opportunities.

The supervision of students to promote understanding of occupation-centred practice requires conscious effort from the educator. This contrasts with *project* or *community development placements* (Overton, Clark and Thomas, 2009) where the focus is often on the delivery of a resource or helping other professionals. Such placements afford students opportunities to develop essential skills for the future workforce, such as skills in communication, collaboration, organisational and time management. It may not, however, promote occupation-centred reasoning skills. This is because within this type of project placement students may follow a project cycle or model from another professional, rather than reasoning for themselves through the occupational therapy process. Being clear about the ultimate purpose of the placement will ensure relevant supports are in place and students experience an appropriate placement variety throughout their education.

FOCAL POINT 3: CHALLENGE PERCEPTIONS

The overarching strategy for the third and last point is for educators to challenge perceptions by:

3.1 Questioning, encouraging and allowing time for students to make sense of their learning
3.2 Allowing learning through 'safe' failure
3.3 Seeking your own supervisory support

FOCAL POINT 3.1: QUESTIONING, ENCOURAGING AND ALLOWING TIME FOR STUDENTS TO MAKE SENSE OF THEIR LEARNING

As students navigate the liminal space of occupation-centred practice they require guidance and support from more experienced colleagues. This guidance and support can take the form of questioning students' evolving understanding of what they are doing, offering reassurance and encouragement, and allowing time for students to explore and try out ideas in authentic situations.

As an educator, you are likely to need to *push* or *press* the students to consider how theory informs their practice (Banks, Bell and Smits, 2000). This includes questioning students, providing gentle feedback and encouragement, and at times being directive to enable them to think through and justify their practice. Example reflective questions proposed by Gibbs (1988) and Johns (2004) are outlined in Table 14.1, with further guidance for educators described in Chapter 11.

Table 14.1 Prompt questions informed by Gibbs's (1988) reflective cycle and Johns's (2004) model of critical reflection

Gibbs (1988)	Johns (2004)
Describe what happened: – What was I thinking? – How did this make me feel? – What was positive about the experience(s)? – What was challenging or uncomfortable about the experience(s)? – What do I think caused or influenced the situation? Why? – What could I have done differently? – What generalisations or learning can I take from this? – How does this tie in with what I have learnt before? – How might I apply this learning in future?	Describe and analyse the situation: – What ultimate purpose was I trying to achieve? – Why did I do what I did? – How effective or successful was it? – How might others have been feeling? – How do I know this? – What knowledge did, or should have informed me? – What was the consequence of using or not using that knowledge? – How could I have handled the situation differently? – How does this connect with my previous experiences? – How do I now feel about this experience?

These approaches resonate with transformative learning theory (Santalucia and Johnson, 2010) in which educators engage students in ongoing dialogue to help them identify gaps and assumptions within their existing knowledge, with the intention of expanding those limits (Rodger et al., 2014). These supervisory techniques can be supplemented with appropriate and timely procedural knowledge (as mentioned in Focal Point 1).

These supervisory techniques are important in both role-established and role-emerging placements. There are, however, some key differences. A feature of role-emerging placements is the greater level of autonomy and the limited potential for direct observation of the students' practice. This means that the 'gentle feedback' can be intensified within the weekly face-to-face supervision, rather than spread throughout the week as might be possible in role-established placements. A weekly intense supervision session can add to the emotional load that students experience. This can, however, also allow students time to formulate and try out their own ideas rather than seeking permission and feedback for each decision they make. Recognising the importance of time and space to try out ideas could also enhance role-established placement experiences.

FOCAL POINT 3.2: ALLOWING LEARNING THROUGH 'SAFE' FAILURE

'Failure' can feel counter-intuitive as an educator as you want to facilitate the students' success during placement. In the initial days and weeks of placement (particularly seen in role-emerging placements), students are often keen to engage in the 'doing' of placement, but with limited reflection and interpretation. While this initial engagement with the placement setting is important, the preliminary intervention ideas the students propose are often not determined on any analysis of assessment information, and are at best a guess based on limited information and experience. Educators are required to bring the students back to the occupational therapy process and support them to reason their interventions appropriately.

Educator guidance needs to be proportionate. It is a useful learning strategy to let students make decisions and try out their ideas, even if you can see that the plan is likely to be unsuccessful. Through trying out ideas students gain confidence as they see the results of their input and can learn from their mistakes in a controlled and supervised environment (Evans and Guile, 2012). The value of this 'positive risk-taking' approach has been described by Slade (2009) as an opportunity to reflect and learn from each new experience and the consequences of actions undertaken. Enabling students to discover for themselves why a course of action is unsuccessful (as opposed to telling them it may fail before they attempt the action) facilitates students' learning and new understandings of their practice.

To facilitate the positive risk-taking approach, you need to withhold some of your concerns with the plan of action from the students to allow them to discover for themselves the strengths and weaknesses of their proposed intervention. This strategy reflects a coaching approach (as mentioned in Focal Point 1), where students are guided to discover their own solutions through questioning from the educator, acting on their understanding of a situation and reflecting on the outcomes (Graham et al., 2017).

You need to be comfortable with giving students the level of freedom to try things out for themselves, whilst ensuring that risks to the student and client(s) are acceptable. You may need to explain your intentions to clients or others within the setting so that they understand it is a learning opportunity for the students. There is a potential risk that clients and others in the setting see the students' slower progress and the 'wrong turns' they make and consider them a reflection on occupational therapy as a profession. This potential needs particular consideration in role-emerging settings where the occupational therapy students are the only experience the clients or service have of occupational therapy. Careful management of expectations here is important.

FOCAL POINT 3.3: SEEKING YOUR OWN SUPERVISORY SUPPORT

Getting your own supervisory support from a peer or mentor is recommended to develop your own skills as well as prevent 'burn out' from the emotional 'roller-coaster' of the placement. Educators are at times required to cope with their own reactions and concerns regarding students' performance, whilst dealing with the students' fluctuating emotions. Discussions with peers (other educators) can provide encouragement and reassurance. This is consistent with the concept of a having a *critical friend* or *critical colleague* (Stenhouse, 1975) as a person who can facilitate the development of reflective and learning capacities of the educator in a supportive, cooperative manner (Kember et al., 1997).

IMPACT OF THE PRACTICE CONTEXT

Within the PLUS Framework (Figure 14.2), student learning and the three Focal Points for educators are surrounded by the practice and university contexts. Practice learning is influenced by the external enablers and constraints of processes, organisational procedures and the culture of both contexts. The different structures of role-emerging and role-established placements also impact on learning opportunities and the knowledge students create and draw upon.

As students are newcomers to the practice setting, they need to become acquainted with the activities, language and the way the setting is organised. This has been described by Lave and Wenger (1991) as "legitimate peripheral participation" (p. 27), where novices undertake peripheral activities to establish themselves within the community of practice. The educator (or on-site supervisor in role-emerging placements) is critical in facilitating access to these peripheral activities. These activities could include introducing students to those staff members and clients who would be open to working with them, making time during meetings for students to contribute and supporting students to successfully navigate the social context of the setting (see Chapter 5). This can be necessary as students are not always universally welcomed by all staff. At times, students can be considered time-consuming for busy staff members and an inconvenience to an already crowded practice setting (Dancza, 2015).

Understanding the different forms of knowledge created and used by students on role-emerging and role-established placements can help us as educators to scaffold students' learning experiences and support the development of professional identity. In the study by Dancza (2015), students reflected that the role-emerging placement was significantly different from their previous role-established placement experiences; it was not simply another experiential learning opportunity. The differences may be partly explained by the shift in balance between the types of knowledge students used and created due to the placement context.

Billett (2010, p. 102) described professional knowledge in three categories: "dispositional knowledge" (values and attitudes of the learner); "domain-specific conceptual knowledge" (facts, concepts, theories); and "domain-specific procedural knowledge" (the processes and procedures).

Dispositional and *conceptual knowledge* can be considered available to all students, whether on role-established or role-emerging placements, as they are derived from university learning and students' previous experiences. Dispositional knowledge includes the students' attitudes towards learning, such as how they critically appraise their work and use reflections to apply new perspectives to their practice. Conceptual knowledge includes knowing about occupational therapy models (such as the OTIPM, Fisher, 2009; CMOP-E , Townsend and Polatajko, 2007; the MOHO , Kielhofner, 2008) and frames of reference (such as the Four Quadrant Model of Facilitated Learning, Greber, Ziviani and Rodger, 2007). Students commence role-established or role-emerging placements with similar exposure to, and experience with, these forms of knowledge.

The availability of *procedural knowledge*, however, differs between role-established and role-emerging placements. Procedural knowledge within occupational therapy could be considered the assessment procedures, documentation formats and standard practices for intervention (such as provision of assistive equipment or classroom-based approaches) (Schell and Schell, 2008). This type of knowledge may be consolidated only within the practice context, despite students having been exposed to many of these processes and practices in a more simulated or hypothetical learning environment at university.

In the study by Dancza (2015), students described learning on their role-established placements as concentrated on procedural knowledge which they acquired in the setting through modelling their behaviour on an occupational therapy educator. Little time was reportedly given to understanding and applying dispositional knowledge (critically appraising what they were doing) or conceptual knowledge (using theory to guide practice).

This all changed on their role-emerging placement when there were no set procedures to follow. Students relied on their own thinking and reflection along with occupational therapy theory to guide their practice (i.e. *dispositional* and *conceptual knowledge*). Additional guidance such as interactive educational resources complemented placement learning and encouraged students to consolidate their professional identity (Dancza, 2015).

IMPACT OF THE UNIVERSITY CONTEXT

The university context also has a profound influence on the students' learning during placements. It is through curriculum content and scaffolding of knowledge and skills throughout the programme that the importance of occupation-centred practice is articulated and reinforced. The university also dictates the placement timing and structure, and expectations to undertake role-emerging, role-established or project (community development) placements.

Particularly for **role-emerging placements**, the time commitments for long-arm supervisors includes face-to-face supervision as well as remote contact. In the study by Dancza (2015), on average long-arm supervisors spent around one day per week in supervisory tasks per placement setting. This time was spread across the week (rather than in a single block) as students were dependent on timely feedback before they could progress their work. During the second half of the placement the time required of long-arm supervisors increased as students produced more work which required reviewing. This was because students were more productive as they gained greater understanding of their role and settled into their placement tasks. Due to the commitment required by the university and the resource intensity of the placements, role-emerging placements should be critically considered by university programmes and adequately resourced to ensure quality learning opportunities which promote the development of professional identity.

For **role-established placements**, the support of the educator (often an occupational therapist in the setting) is vital. Ensuring that students experience occupation-centred practice requires educators to feel confident in articulating their own theory to practice links. This can be supported through the provision of educator-training programmes by the university which focus on theory and reasoning, with ongoing guidance by the university to support educators during the placement as required.

Project (community development) placements can require a different focus for educators. Navigating learning thresholds of occupation-centred practice is less likely to be the primary emphasis in supervision. Thus, it may be that educators can support students in a way which is less resource intensive.

Potential resources which could be developed within the university context to support students and educators in placement learning include:

- The introduction of frameworks such as the PLUS Framework that highlight the critical features of supervisory practices to ensure efficient use of these precious resources
- Scheduling of student group reflective discussions at key time points during the placement (i.e. immediately prior to placement, around the midpoint of placement and after placement) to facilitate student learning and possibly save time for educators. Exploration of how to do this using a mixture of face-to-face and online platforms could enable a group of students to present cases and engage in theory-practice discussions with one educator.

CHAPTER SUMMARY

This chapter has introduced the link between practice learning and the development of professional identity. It explored the idea of transformative learning theories including threshold concepts, unpacked some of the complexities of practice learning, and presented the PLUS Framework. The PLUS Framework provides a fulcrum between established structures and process for students to follow and the requirement for students to facilitate their own learning. Professional identity development is a key outcome of practice learning. It requires an occupation-centred curriculum to precede it, as well as opportunities for professional conversations for students to consolidate their learning and sense of professional identity.

REFERENCES

Ashby SE, Adler J, Herbert L (2016) 'An exploratory international study into occupational therapy students' perceptions of professional identity'. *Australian Occupational Therapy Journal, 63*(4), 233–243.

Ashby SE, Ryan S, Gray M, James C (2013) 'Factors that influence the professional resilience of occupational therapists in mental health practice'. *Australian Occupational Therapy Journal, 60*(2), 110–119.

Banks S, Bell E, Smits E (2000) 'Integration tutorials and seminars: Examining the integration of academic and fieldwork learning by student occupational therapists'. *Canadian Journal of Occupational Therapy, 67*(2), 93–100.

Billett S (2010) 'Emerging perspectives of work: Implications for university teaching and learning'. In: J Higgs, D Fish, I Goulter, S Loftus, J Reid, F Trede, eds, *Education for future practice*. Rotterdam, The Netherlands: Sense Publishers, pp. 97–112.

Chaiklin S (2003) 'The zone of proximal development in Vygotsky's analysis of learning and instruction'. In: A Kozulin, B Gindis, V Ageyev, S Miller, eds, *Vygotsky's educational theory and practice in cultural context*. Cambridge, UK: Cambridge University, pp. 39–64.

Cousin G (2006) 'An introduction to threshold concepts'. *Planet, 17*, 4–5.

Dancza KM (2015) *Structure and uncertainty: The 'just right' balance for occupational therapy student learning on role-emerging placements in schools*. Doctor of Philosophy, The University of Queensland, Queensland, Australia.

Dancza KM, Copley J, Rodger S, Moran M (2016) 'The development of a theory-informed workbook as an additional support for students on role-emerging placements'. *British Journal of Occupational Therapy, 79*(4), 235–243.

Dreyfus H, Dreyfus S (1986) *Mind over machine: The power of human intuition and expertise in the era of the computer*. New York: The Free Press.

Du Toit S, Wilkinson AC (2011) 'Promoting an appreciation for research-related activities: The role of occupational identity'. *British Journal of Occupational Therapy*, 74(10), 489–492.

Evans K, Guile D (2012) 'Putting different forms of knowledge to work in practice'. In: J Higgs, R Barnett, S Billett, M Hutchings, F Trede, eds, *Practice-based education: Perspectives and strategies*. Rotterdam, The Netherlands: Sense Publishers, pp. 113–130.

Fisher AG (2009) *Occupational therapy intervention process model: A model for planning and implementing top-down, client centred, and occupation-based interventions*. Fort Collins, CO: Three Star Press.

Fortune T, Kennedy-Jones M (2014) 'Occupation and its relationship with health and wellbeing: The threshold concept for occupational therapy'. *Australian Occupational Therapy Journal*, 61(5), 293–298.

Gibbs G (1988) *Learning by doing: A guide to teaching and learning methods*. Oxford, UK: Oxford Polytechnic.

Graham F, Rodger S, Kennedy-Behr A (2017) 'Occupational Performance Coaching (OPC): Enabling caregivers' and children's occupational performance'. In: S Rodger, A Kennedy-Behr, eds, *Occupation-centred practice with children: A practical guide for occupational therapists*. 2nd edn. West Sussex, UK: Wiley-Blackwell, pp. 209–232.

Greber C, Ziviani J, Rodger S (2007) 'The Four Quadrant Model of Facilitated Learning: A clinically based action research project'. *Australian Occupational Therapy Journal*, 54(2), 149–152.

Health and Care Professions Council (2013) *Standards of proficiency Occupational Therapists*. Great Britain: Health and Care Professions Council.

Hooper B, King R, Wood W, Bilics AR, Gupta J (2013) 'An international systemic mapping review of educational approaches and teaching methods in occupational therapy'. *British Journal of Occupational Therapy*, 76, 9–22.

Huggins D (2016) 'Enhancing nursing students' education by coaching mentors'. *Nursing Management*, 23(1), 30–32.

Ikiugu MN (2012) 'Use of theoretical conceptual practice models by occupational therapists in the US: A pilot survey'. *International Journal of Therapy and Rehabilitation*, 19(11), 629–637.

Johns C (2004) *Becoming a reflective practitioner.* Oxford, UK: Wiley Blackwell.

Kember D, Ha T, Lam B, Lee A, NG S, Yan L, Yum J (1997) 'The diverse role of the critical friend in supporting educational action research projects'. *Education Action Research,* 5(3), 463–481.

Kessler D, Graham F (2015) 'The use of coaching in occupational therapy: An integrative review'. *Australian Occupational Therapy Journal,* 62(3), 160–176.

Kielhofner G (2008) *A model of human occupation: Theory and application.* 4th edn. Baltimore, MD: Lippincott Williams & Wilkins.

Kolb DA (1984) *Experiential learning: Experience as the source of learning and development.* London: Prentice-Hall.

Kronenberg F, Pollard N, Sakellariou D, eds (2011) *Occupational therapies without borders – Volume 2: Towards an ecology of occupation-based practices.* 2nd edn. Oxford, UK: Churchill Livingstone.

Lave J, Wenger E (1991) *Situated learning: Legitimate peripheral participation.* Cambridge, UK: Cambridge University Press.

Lindquist I, Engardt M, Garnham L, Poland F, Richardson B (2006) 'Physiotherapy students' professional identity on the edge of working life'. *Medical Teacher,* 28(3), 270–276.

Meyer JHF, Land R (2003) 'Threshold concepts and troublesome knowledge: Linkages to ways of thinking and practicing within disciplines'. In: C Rust, ed, *Improving student learning – Ten years on.* Edinburgh, UK: OCSLD, pp. 1–15.

Meyer JHF, Land R (2005) 'Threshold concepts and troublesome knowledge (2): Epistemological considerations and a conceptual framework for teaching and learning'. *Higher Education,* 49, 373–388.

Mezirow J (1997) 'Transformative Learning: Theory to Practice'. *New Directions for Adult and Continuing Education,* 74, 5–12, doi:10.1002/ace.7401

Mezirow J (2000) 'Learning to think like an adult: Core concepts of transformative theory'. In: J Mezirow, ed, *Learning as transformation.* San Francisco, CA: Jossey-Bass, pp. 3–34.

Molineux M (2011) 'Standing firm on shifting sands'. *New Zealand Journal of Occupational Therapy,* 58(1), 21–28.

Morrison T, Robertson L (2016) 'New graduates' experience of evidence-based practice: An action research study'. *British Journal of Occupational Therapy,* 79(1), 42–48.

Overton A, Clark M, Thomas Y (2009) 'A review of non-traditional occupational therapy practice placement education: A focus on role-emerging and project placements'. *British Journal of Occupational Therapy, 72*(7), 294–301.

Rodger S, Thomas Y, Greber C, Broadbridge J, Edwards A, Newton J and Lyons M (2014) 'Attributes of excellence in practice educators: The perspectives of Australian occupational therapy students'. *Australian Occupational Therapy Journal,* 61(3), 159–167. doi:10.1111/1440-1630.12096

Rodger S, Turpin M (2011) 'Using threshold concepts to transform entry level curricula'. *Research and development in higher education: Higher education on the edge, Higher Education Research and Development Society of Australasia,* 4–7 July 2011, pp. 263–274.

Royal College of Occupational Therapists (2008) *Standards for education: Pre-registration education standards.* London, UK: Royal College of Occupational Therapists.

Royal College of Occupational Therapists (2017) *Career development framework: Guiding principles for occupational therapy.* London, UK: Royal College of Occupational Therapists.

Sabari JS (1985) 'Professional socialisation: Implications for occupational therapy education'. *American Journal of Occupational Therapy, 39*(2), 96–102.

Santalucia SE, Johnson CR (2010) 'Transformative learning: Facilitating growth and change through fieldwork'. *OT Practice, 15*(19), CE1–CE8.

Schell BAB, Schell JW, eds (2008) *Clinical and professional reasoning in occupational therapy.* Philadelphia, PA: Walters Kluwer/Lippincott, Williams & Wilkins.

Schon DA (1983) *The reflective practitioner: How professionals think in action.* New York, USA: Basic Books Inc.

Slade M (2009) *Personal recovery and mental illness: A guide for mental health professionals.* Cambridge: Cambridge University Press.

Stenhouse L (1975) *An introduction to curriculum research and development.* UK: Heinemann.

Tanner B (2011) 'Threshold concepts in practice education: Perceptions of practice educators'. *British Journal of Occupational Therapy, 74*(9), 427–434.

Towns E, Ashby S (2014) 'The influence of practice educators on occupational therapy students' understanding of the practical applications of theoretical knowledge: A phenomenological study into student experiences of practice education'. *Australian Occupational Therapy Journal, 61*(5), 344–352.

Townsend E, Polatajko HJ, eds (2007) *Enabling occupation II: Advancing an occupational therapy vision for health, well-being and justice through occupation.* Ottawa, ON: CAOT Publications ACE.

Turner A (2011) 'The Elizabeth Casson Memorial lecture 2011: Occupational therapy – A profession in adolescence?'. *British Journal of Occupational Therapy,* 74(7), 314–322.

Unsworth CA (2001) 'The clinical reasoning of novice and expert occupational therapists'. *Scandinavian Journal of Occupational Therapy, 8,* 163–173.

Volkert A (2017) *The Development of professional identity in new graduate occupational therapists.* Professional Doctorate in Education, Leeds Beckett University.

Vygotsky L (1978) *Mind in society.* Cambridge, MA: Harvard University Press.

Wilding C, Whiteford G (2007) 'Occupation and occupational therapy: Knowledge paradigms and everyday practice'. *Australian Occupational Therapy Journal, 54*(3), 185–193.

World Federation of Occupational Therapists (2002) *Minimum standards for the education of occupational therapists.* Geneva: World Federation Occupational Therapists.

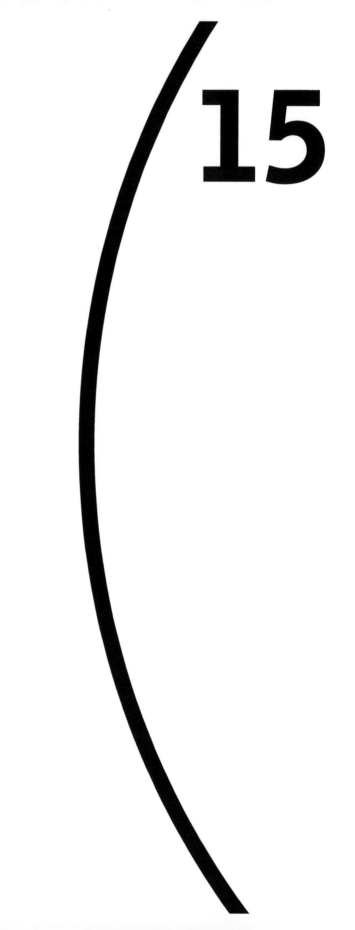

15

CHAPTER 15
CASE STUDIES IN PLACEMENT SETTINGS WITHOUT AN ESTABLISHED OCCUPATIONAL THERAPY ROLE (ROLE-EMERGING)

Karina Dancza, Ann Kennedy-Behr and Caroline Hui

INTENDED CHAPTER OUTCOMES

By the end of this chapter, readers will have an overview of:

- How this book may be used in role-emerging placement settings in different parts of the world
- Some of the successes and challenges faced in implementing an occupation-centred practice experience for students
- Practical tips for using this resource in a range of contexts

INTRODUCTION

Implementing an occupation-centred approach in practice is an exciting, yet challenging prospect. Using the Occupational Therapy Intervention Process Model (OTIPM; Fisher, 2009) as the structure followed in this book has enabled the practical (and consistent) application of these ideas in a range of settings.

The first case study focuses on the original doctoral research which evaluated student learning of role-emerging placements in school settings in the United Kingdom. Over the five year period of the doctoral study, four action research cycles enabled a draft of this book to be developed and evaluated. This case study describes the use of the draft book and strategies that educators from Canterbury Christ Church University employed during their supervision sessions with students to promote critical thinking and reasoning.

The second case study was developed at the University of the Sunshine Coast, Australia. It outlines the use of the occupation-centred approach in an international role-emerging placement context. Students were supported during their placement in Vanuatu whilst being supervised from their Australian university. It outlines the aspects of the book which were directly applied to the placement along with a description of how it was contextualised.

The third case study is based on the experiences of implementing the book in school-based practice in Canada. It was used with two students from l'Université de Sherbrooke in their last placement before graduation. This case study describes the use of the book in the role-emerging setting with a long-arm (off-site) supervisor.

CASE STUDY 1: UNITED KINGDOM SCHOOL-BASED ROLE-EMERGING PLACEMENT (KARINA DANCZA)

CONTEXT

The development of this book began from my own (Karina Dancza) experiences supervising students undertaking role-emerging placements in primary school settings in the United Kingdom. The students and I both experienced anxiety in implementing an occupational therapy process in a school which remained focused on the children's school occupations. My investigation of what strategies supported the students' learning during their role-emerging placement turned into my PhD study and resulted in the development and evaluation of this book (Dancza, Copley, Rodger and Moran, 2016). It was through a process of action research, where changes to the book were made and then evaluated with the next group of students, that this book evolved. Four action research cycles involved 14 students and 11 educators who contributed to the research. The following sections highlight some of the most challenging, although rewarding experiences when implementing this approach.

SUPERVISION WHICH FOCUSED ON UNPACKING, EXPLORING AND ACKNOWLEDGING LEARNING

During the research, students and educators consistently discussed their experiences of supervision. In previous role-established placements, the students reflected that the focus of 'traditional' supervision was somewhat perfunctory and primarily involved monitoring their timetable and completion of administrative processes, such as checking paperwork relating to their learning objectives, reflections and timesheets. By contrast during the role-emerging placement, students appreciated how supervision made them 'think deeply'. As I was not in the situation with the students, I needed their detailed descriptions of what happened to know how to guide them. Therefore, supervision time was spent *unpacking, exploring* and *acknowledging* students' progress.

During the research all long-arm supervisors used the book structure and the OTIPM as a key guide. However, we found that we 'instinctively' developed our own supervisory techniques. I don't recall this being a conscious decision initially, although it did become more apparent because the research process prompted reflection and critical discussions.

A common discussion we had as long-arm supervisors was how uncomfortable we felt at times when we needed to challenge students to think deeply about how their proposed assessment and intervention ideas linked with an occupational therapy theory or practice model. It felt like we were making situations more complex for students as we wanted them to understand *why* they might do something, rather than simply telling them what we thought they should do.

One of my key strategies was to bring the students back to theory and the occupational therapy process at each supervision session (hence the reason I have included the OTIPM diagram at the start of each chapter in Part II). I also tried to make my own reasoning explicit to the students. This required considerable conscious effort and I did often ask myself if I was overwhelming the students.

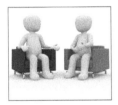

PRACTICAL TIPS

1   As students were explaining what happened during supervision, I tried to link their examples with an occupational therapy model or theory. Repetition and reflection were key to this process.
2   Throughout the supervision, I gave students the opportunity to pause and write down any ideas or learning moments. I also kept in mind that students would need many of these points reinforced during the placement to consolidate their learning.

USING THIS BOOK AND THE OTIPM

Frequent comments were made by educators and students about this book's usefulness in guiding them through the uncertainties of practice learning. Some students referred to the book as "long-arm supervision without the long-arm supervisor".

The book was seen by students and educators as a way of offering some certainty through the explanation of the occupational therapy process, with illustrative examples of tasks they could do to enact this process. Students could also refer to it when they needed to, outside of the face-to-face supervision sessions. A few on-site supervisors were also interested in the book as it offered them background to the students' work and helped them know what was expected of the students in their placement.

Students discussed how they relied on the book as an authoritative source of information. They did describe, however, how unsettled they were when the long-arm supervisor recommended a different course of action from that presented in the book, as it led the students back into unknown territory.

While some students referred to the book throughout placement, others found it helpful at specific time points. Prior to placement and during the first few weeks, students particularly valued the explicit links which were made between university learning and the placement context, suggestions for specific reading and prompts regarding role explanations to various stakeholders. Pleasingly, some students reported that, towards the second half of placement, they relied less on the book as their own reasoning developed. On further exploration, however, this may have been as the book was less directive about possible intervention strategies as each situation is unique. Students still needed to justify what they were doing, so were prompted to continue using the OTIPM to support their reasoning.

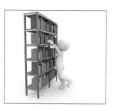

PRACTICAL TIPS
....

1   Students may need prompting to access information when relevant during placement. For example, they may need explicit reminding of the guidance offered in this book or tools they have used in their university programme (such as how to run a group, risk assessment tools, communication skills etc.).
2   When the students need something which is different from the book, such as a different report format or way of prioritising occupational needs, discuss with them what is required and why, so they can understand and apply flexibility in their reasoning.

LIMITED FACE-TO-FACE CONTACT WITH STUDENTS

The structure of the role-emerging placement afforded unique opportunities for me as an academic to retain important connections with practice. It did, however, also present a range of challenges that were reported by all long-arm supervisors involved in my study.

Specifically, we felt responsible for the students' learning. However, we could not guide the students through this learning by modelling relevant skills, such as interview or assessment techniques in the way we would have done had we been supervising them on-site all the time. Instead, students were required to explain to us the work they had been doing between supervision sessions in sufficient detail so that we could check their reasoning and offer guidance for the next steps.

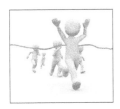

PRACTICAL TIPS

1   In the first few weeks of placement it is useful to undertake an observation
    alongside the students of a priority occupation in the placement setting (e.g.
    a sport lesson, writing activity in class, mealtime, play in the playground). This
    offers students the opportunity to observe how an experienced occupational
    therapist interacts with the school staff members and children and compare their
    observations.
2   Going with students on a pre-placement visit is a useful way of modelling and
    guiding students in their interactions with placement staff members and clients.

BALANCING LEARNING OPPORTUNITIES WITH PROVIDING A SERVICE FOR THE SETTING

Our discussions amongst the long-arm supervisors often focused on how there was a
compromise needed between giving students the space and time for learning (sometimes
from their mistakes) and providing an effective and responsive service to the school. The
time needed for students to reason through their observations and assessments to instigate
interventions appeared to some teachers to result in a significant delay to the service the
students were providing to the school.

To facilitate the balance between student learning and service delivery, I and other
educators purposefully used a range of supervisory strategies from being *directive and
explicit* about what the students should do, to being *non-directive and more of a facilitator*
to enable the students to determine his/her own course of action.

Giving students space to try out their ideas and discover the successes and consequences
was an important learning strategy for students. This did, however, cause me and some
other educators considerable anxiety. We needed to be comfortable to let students
continue with sometimes less-than-optimal plans so that they could see the flaws in their
approach for themselves and learn from those experiences. To make these decisions we had
to consider the impact of the students' actions (particularly as we were not there all the
time) and calculate whether it would not cause harm or unnecessary delay to the school.
This often required us as educators to talk through these scenarios together and consider
the risks to reassure ourselves we were doing the right thing.

With the need to independently develop their own roles within the school, students were
at times unsure of themselves and would repeatedly check their planning of an assessment
or intervention strategy with me and postpone its execution. Students appeared hesitant
to try out their plans and wanted to gather more assessment information to answer all

their questions before they proceeded. I needed to *push the students out of their comfort zone* through consistent (but supportive) pressure to initiate, complete and critically reflect on what they were *doing* (not just thinking about doing). This was reported by students and other educators to be a necessary, although often difficult, aspect of the role-emerging placement and an uncomfortable part of supervision.

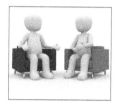

PRACTICAL TIPS

1   Where possible, give the students space to try something out and see the results for themselves. Leaving students to think through a decision can provide valuable learning opportunities.
2   This approach, however, does take time and open discussions may be needed with the placement setting to balance the needs of the students with those of the setting.

APPLYING OCCUPATION-CENTRED PRINCIPLES IN PRACTICE

The initial challenge I faced which prompted the development of this book and my PhD research was how complex and exhausting it was to support students' practice in a way which centred on occupation. This appeared compounded by feedback from students that they had not explicitly applied theoretical concepts to their practice on previous placements. Some students did report they had used a model on a previous placement, but it had been in the form of an assessment tool or linked with one part of the occupational therapy process (i.e. assessment) but not followed through.

This was further exacerbated at times when some students did not appear to place any importance on the use of theory, perhaps due to their confusion over its relevance to practice. Explicitly applying theory to practice and being able to explain my own reasoning to students was also not always straightforward. I needed to develop confidence in articulating how theoretical concepts informed my practice in the placement setting. Interestingly, some long-arm supervisors chose to share their uncertainties with the students during the supervision sessions to emphasise the complexities and effort (and rewards) involved in using theory in practice.

I believe the wider context of occupational therapy service provision to children in the United Kingdom also had a significant impact on the students' learning. Applying occupation-centred theory to their placement meant that the occupational therapy provision by the students in the school was different from that provided by some local occupational therapy services. At the time of the research, the focus of local services tended to be on reduction of impairment (e.g. implementing motor or sensory programmes), whereas the students were concerned with enabling the children's participation in school occupations.

This differing perspective presented real challenges. For example, when there was an occupational therapist visiting the school from a local service, or a programme recommended by an occupational therapist was left with the school to carry out, the school staff members asked for the students to become involved. Potential for conflict arose when there were differences between my guidance of the students and the recommendations of local occupational therapists.

I (as well as other educators) felt a responsibility to highlight the differences between occupation-centred and impairment-focussed practice to the students. We thought it was important for students to have the links between theory and practice made explicit. In doing this, however, I felt like I was discrediting the approach of my professional colleagues. I found this a particularly uncomfortable position. In one of my most challenging (although thankfully rare) situations, one where I felt the child and teacher were being placed at risk by attempting to implement a sensory-motor programme, I had to discuss my concerns directly with the school staff member and not leave the responsibility to the students to convey my concern. I then assisted the school to raise the issue directly with the local occupational therapist involved.

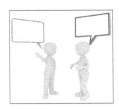

PRACTICAL TIPS

1   Through completing a risk assessment together with students, you can support students to recognise when it is useful for them to take responsibility to raise an issue and when they would benefit from seeing how an experienced occupational therapist does this – both are useful learning opportunities.
2   As an educator, there may be times where you feel it is necessary to challenge current practices. Discussions with the students and, where appropriate, other educators can help clarify the issues and develop strategies to manage these complex situations.

EDUCATORS NEEDING SUPPORT

There is an emotional load associated with supervising students. We, as educators, are required to contain the students' uncertainties as well as manage a delicate balance of challenging and supporting them. We also need to manage the seemingly competing priorities between provision of a service in the setting and the time and space needed for students' learning.

As educators, I feel we have our own support needs. I found the role of supervisor to be one of the most rewarding aspects of student education, but I couldn't have done it without the support of my colleagues. I also needed to be realistic about the time commitments of this role. Seeking my own support, responding to emails, reviewing the students' work, offering telephone feedback or providing reassurance to students and on-site supervisors were all undertaken outside the face-to-face supervision sessions.

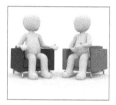

PRACTICAL TIPS

1   Peer support networks for long-arm supervisors can help manage the emotional load associated with role-emerging placements. Having an opportunity to debrief after a supervision session can be helpful to clarify the current situation with the students and the advice/guidance provided.
2   Reflecting with other educators on how students are progressing using learning theories (such as threshold concepts) can help make sense of the fluctuations which may be apparent in the students' understanding of occupational therapy practice and reduce some of the anxieties associated with supervision.

CASE STUDY 2: AUSTRALIA – VANUATU ROLE-EMERGING AND STUDENT-LED PLACEMENTS (ANN KENNEDY-BEHR)

CONTEXT

In Australia, many undergraduate occupational therapy programmes are four-year Bachelor programmes with most large block placements occurring in the third and fourth years of study. At the University of the Sunshine Coast (USC) in Southeast Queensland, students can go on a variety of different placements including rural and remote locations. The various placement opportunities have different supervision models including the traditional apprentice model, role-emerging placements and student-led practice education. At USC, the term 'student-led practice' is used where there may be an established occupational therapy role, however there might not be an on-site occupational therapist.

The initial idea to use the book to support students on placement in Vanuatu (a small island nation in the South Pacific) arose through a combination of my (Ann Kennedy-Behr) wanting to provide the best possible practice education experience for the students and my concern that I was not entirely sure what kind of practice experiences the students would have. Also, with a ratio of one practice educator to six occupational therapy students, I would not always be available and I wanted the students to have an extra resource that they could use.

Dr. Dancza's (2015) original book (the draft version of this current book) was adapted for USC students three times: two iterations for two visits, eight months apart, to Vanuatu and a third iteration which incorporated contextualisation for both domestic and international student-led placements.

The placement on Santo, Vanuatu was classed as role-emerging as there was no established occupational therapy role at the district hospital or within any other service on the island. The island of Santo has a population of approximately 40,000 people, with one large town (where the hospital is located) and many small and remote villages. Some of the villages have small clinics or aid posts, but neither the hospital nor the clinics have any allied health staff. While there are medical and surgical services available at the hospital, rehabilitation services and home visits are not provided.

A brief scoping visit had already been conducted, however there were still many unknowns and it was anticipated that the students and I would potentially be working in health-promotion roles, as well as providing services to clients identified through the existing health-care system. I went with the students to Vanuatu and stayed with them for four weeks of their seven-week placement. The remainder of my support for the students was via email and weekly Skype® internet conferences.

CONTEXTUALISING THE BOOK

The original book was adapted by me in preparation for going to Vanuatu. Changes made included writing a different introduction, including safety information and contact numbers, changing the timeline to suit our placement structure and providing different supplementary readings (such as Pidgeon, 2015). While I was confident that the principles contained in the book could be easily adapted to any setting, I was not sure that students would be able to do this without assistance.

The students were given the book prior to our departure for Vanuatu and asked to familiarise themselves with it. In the first week in Vanuatu I asked all students to complete two chapters (Chapters 5 and 6 in this book) and to consider how they would introduce themselves in this context. In the second adaptation of the book, I provided an example of how students might introduce themselves to clients in Vanuatu. For most of the clients with whom we worked, English was a second or third language and the students gained valuable experience in communicating the purpose of occupational therapy in simple, everyday language. Providing examples to them of how they might do this supported their initial efforts and provided a base that they could build on. My discussions with students went something like this:

"Working in Vanuatu is complex. Occupational therapy is not well known and English is often a second language for other health professionals as well as clients and families. This can impact communication. It is important that you convey what you are going to do in everyday language. For example, 'I am here to help your child play and learn.'

When working with adults, you might choose to focus on typical occupations. For example, 'I am here to help you do the things you need to do, like getting dressed or cooking a meal.'

Since there are only very limited allied health staff on Santo, as occupational therapy students, you will need to consider the whole situation and work on priorities for the person and family. This could mean dealing with pressing safety concerns (such as teaching carers to transfer a person safely so they can get out of bed and move around the house and community in a wheelchair) or working together with people on adapting the environment to enable occupations (such as mealtimes, play etc.)."

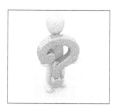

PRACTICAL TIPS

1   Before using the book with students, consider how it fits with your context and whether any supplementary information (e.g. specific readings) needs to be added. The 'Educator examples here' prompts (see Appendix 1.1) offer a helpful starting point and you can continue developing examples throughout the placement.
2   Adapt the placement timeline (as suggested in Chapter 5) to reflect the length of the students' placement and how you anticipate they will be proceeding through it. This can help students see that in a role-emerging placement they need more 'thinking' time as they cannot follow the established processes or model their practice on an occupational therapist in the setting.

USING THE BOOK IN SUPERVISION

During the students' seven weeks in Vanuatu I directed them to read specific chapters. I found that without direction the students tended not to read the book, but when they did they found it very useful. This was similarly reported by the practice educators for students on domestic placements. I used the book as 'homework', asking the students to read specific chapters by certain dates and then we reviewed their learning during supervision. This provided a formal structure for the supervision sessions and helped the students make the connection between theory and practice.

Using the peer feedback form in Chapter 12 was particularly useful. I asked students to observe one of their peers and provide formal feedback using the suggested structure. I instructed them not to share the contents of the peer evaluation with me, but rather to write a reflection on the process and share that. The reflections indicated the depth of learning and their progression towards becoming professionals. I also asked the students to write a reflection on the process of evaluating their peers. Some of the reflections indicated that this was the first time the student had tried to see themselves from someone else's perspective. The reflections gave the students space to identify knowledge that they had already internalised and provided an opportunity to reflect on their own skill development.

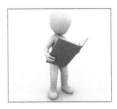

PRACTICAL TIPS
....

1   Ask students to complete specific pages from the book by a certain date. Given the intensity of practice education and differing learning styles, be prepared that not all students will be self-directed in reading the book.
2   The activities in the book act as useful prompts for students to reflect on their practice. Sharing these activities with their peer or in supervision is a useful learning strategy and they can be used as a basis to complete required placement reflections and learning objectives.

DOCUMENTATION

The students found Chapter 9 on documentation very beneficial and needed little support in adapting the examples to their situation. The example of the occupational therapy report in Chapter 9 was used as a model by all students to write their final reports. I added information on assessment to this chapter, noting that most formal occupational therapy assessments have been developed in Europe and North America and cautioned that they were not necessarily appropriate for use in other settings.

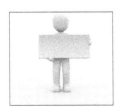

PRACTICAL TIPS
....

1   If you have a documentation style you would like students to use, or one that is required by the placement setting, provide an example of this for students to follow.
2   If you are supporting students on a role-emerging placement, you can develop a bank of examples as you return to the same placement setting. Ask students' permission to use their work as examples for the next student group.

REMOTE DIGITAL SUPERVISION AND LIMITED ON-SITE RESOURCES

I returned to Australia for the final three weeks of placement and was therefore very much a long-arm supervisor. Supervision was conducted via Skype and email, which was challenging as internet access was sporadic and often restricted to when students were in the main hospital, but overall it worked well. Having a book where we could quite literally be 'on the same page' helped me support the students and seemed to give them confidence that they were still being supported, albeit from a distance.

Students from the first trip to Vanuatu commented that the book was particularly useful given the limited internet access. While they had been accustomed to using the internet as a resource for many of their queries, in Vanuatu, as in some regional and remote areas of Australia, internet access was not always reliable or of sufficient speed to download the necessary resources. Students used the book with the examples as a way of supplementing their knowledge and supporting their learning.

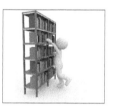

PRACTICAL TIPS

1   Alert students to the fact that they might not always have internet access for their research and that the book contains many resources which can support them.
2   For long-arm supervisors, asking students to turn to a specific page during the supervision session may further help the students feel supported and make the supervision feel more 'real'.

CASE STUDY 3: CANADA ROLE-EMERGING SCHOOL-BASED PLACEMENT (CAROLINE HUI)

CONTEXT

In Quebec, Canada, Dr. Dancza's draft book (2015) was initially used with two Université de Sherbrooke occupational therapy students during their final seven-week placement. At the Université de Sherbrooke, students are enrolled in a four-year professional Master's program with six placements ranging from direct supervision to long-arm supervision. The students' placement was in a role-emerging setting in an elementary (primary) school with a long-arm (off-site) occupational therapy supervisor, who was an educator from the university.

In Canada, occupational therapy services for children are not mandated and each province differs in terms of the services it provides to school pupils. In the Province of Quebec, few school boards offer occupational therapy services. Occupational therapists had not worked in this particular school before. Thus, many of the teachers with whom the students collaborated and worked did not know about the role of occupational therapy.

Being relatively new to student supervision and having only one long-arm supervision experience in the past, I (Caroline Hui) was motivated to use this book to support student learning more effectively. I had the benefit of being supported by Dr. Kennedy-Behr (author of the second case study) and I could ask her advice throughout the placement. Similar to Dr. Kennedy-Behr's example, I also changed the timeline to match the students' placement schedule, and added references on self-regulation programs and occupational performance coaching.

Although Université de Sherbrooke is a French university and the placement was in French schools, these students were bilingual, so the book was not translated into French.

USING THE OTIPM WHEN IT IS NOT THE STUDENTS' USUAL OCCUPATIONAL THERAPY MODEL

At Université de Sherbrooke the primary model students use in the occupational therapy program is the Canadian Practice Process Framework (CPPF, associated with the Canadian Model of Occupational Performance and Engagement – see Chapter 2; Townsend and Polatajko, 2013). As students were following this book during this placement, this was the first time they used the OTIPM to guide their practice.

Early during placement a diagram of both the CPPF and OTIPM was presented to the students, and the differences and similarities were identified and discussed. Although one student felt that the OTIPM's diagram was visually more complex than the CPPF's diagram, both students were open to using another model. The students reflected how they found the OTIPM to be more comprehensive than the CPPF they were familiar with, as the OTIPM included different approaches for intervention. Overall, they reported that using a different model was not difficult as the OTIPM and examples in the book showed them where they were in each step of the occupational therapy process.

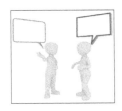

PRACTICAL TIPS

1   If you are using the book in a situation where students are unfamiliar with the OTIPM, spend time discussing similarities and differences between the models. Chapter 2 offers a brief overview of some of the common occupational therapy models and a comparison between them as a potential starting point.
2   If you are not familiar with the OTIPM, with some pre-reading and preparation you can learn how to implement it alongside the students during the placement.

SUPPORTING STUDENTS' REASONING WHEN THE LONG-ARM SUPERVISOR IS NOT ALWAYS THERE

One of the tools the university suggests using during supervision is a student logbook. A logbook is used by students to write a description of a case or situation which occurred during the day, the student's analysis of what happened, and what they might do differently or not for next time. The students were encouraged to reflect on what was important or significant for them each day. At times, they used the activities and prompts in the book as a basis for these reflections.

The students and I followed the book chapters (in Part II) to structure our supervision meetings (either on-site or via Google™ Hangouts). Although I was based off-site, I felt that the logbook reflections in conjunction with discussion on the activities they completed in the book provided me with specific information on their placement experiences and reasoning skills.

The reflections and activities within the book also supported students to learn from their peer and develop their reasoning without me being there all the time to guide them. Students worked together and could provide peer support to each other. For example, as both students did observations using the occupational performance analysis (Chapter 4), they could compare the details of their assessments. This lead to a discussion on how behaviours in the classroom can be interpreted differently as students separated out what they observed from what they thought was potentially causing the challenges (expressed in the OTIPM as clarifying or interpreting the reasons for the client's problems of occupational performance – Chapter 11). Students could then identify multiple possibilities for intervention. This reflected the needs of the teachers and pupils in the classroom and enabled the students to tailor their approach based on their own reasoning and client-centred principles. Additionally, the Six Thinking Hats (De Bono, 1985) exercise in Chapter 7 was useful to view each of their goals from different perspectives.

Without having a supervisor on-site to guide them all the time, the students used these activities to independently develop their thinking skills. Students also collaborated with the school teachers more effectively since they had analysed what they were doing from many perspectives and could see what obstacles needed to be overcome to help the children achieve their goals. One student reported that the Six Thinking Hats activity helped her visualise different options and anticipate the reactions of key players, such as the teachers and children.

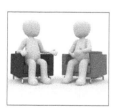

PRACTICAL TIPS
....

1   The book can offer a useful structure for supervision sessions. The activities are particularly helpful for exploring students' reasoning.

2   Encourage students to discuss their completed activities with their peer before
    supervision sessions or write their thoughts in a reflective logbook. This enables
    students to articulate their reasoning and rehearse what they wish to cover in the
    limited supervision time.

STUDENTS' NEED FOR STRUCTURE AND EXAMPLES

Students were given the book four weeks before the placement (due to the timing
of vacation) and both read it in the week prior to the start of the placement. Both
students reported that the book was very useful and identified that the section in
Chapter 5 on 'Planning your learning' was their favourite. This activity helped them
to reflect on their skills and to identify their strengths and areas to improve. This
was particularly helpful as students were required to complete something similar in a
Learning Contract (a mandatory contract used by the university as a tool to enhance
communication and collaboration between student and educator). Although the
Learning Contract must be completed, it does not offer specific guidance or examples
to help students elaborate on their learning strengths and weaknesses. The book,
however, suggests desired attributes and provides reflective questions to help their
thinking. One student stated that it made her question what type of occupational
therapist she wanted to be.

In terms of workload, students did not feel that reading and completing the activities
in the book added substantially to their tasks. Students could see the relevance of the
activities in assisting them during their placement and felt they required minimal extra
time to complete. In addition, the students reported that certain questions and examples
helped validate their own thinking and actions.

As the placement unfolded, the students used the book less frequently than at the
beginning. They reported feeling more confident in their role and had a clear direction
of the process. Whilst the increased confidence was commended, students still needed to
follow the occupational therapy process to the end of their placement, and not go off on
their own track. Students therefore needed more encouragement to use the book in the
latter stages of their placement to ensure that their reasoning was sound and that they
were guided by theory in their intervention and evaluation procedures.

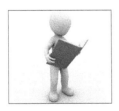

PRACTICAL TIPS

1   Consider the placement paperwork that students are required to complete. Help
    the students to see the connections between the activities in the book and the
    reflections and learning objectives in their university paperwork. These learning aids
    need not be mutually exclusive and students may use one to inform the other.

2   Despite the students' increasing confidence, the educator needs to encourage students to continue following the occupational therapy process until the end of placement. This can be done by referring to the book and OTIPM and continuing to elicit students' reasoning with reflective questions.

LONG-ARM (OFF-SITE) SUPERVISOR'S NEED FOR STRUCTURE AND EXAMPLES

In role-emerging placements where uncertainty is rife and anxiety amongst students is common, using the book provided students with an extra resource and reassurance. It also provided me (their long-arm supervisor) with a structure for the supervision I offered. As I was using the book for the first time I had to familiarise myself with it during the placement. I was not sure what to expect from the students but was pleased with their enthusiasm to read the book and complete the activities. On my part, it required more preparation than I initially expected, but with practice I think it will become easier to incorporate into the supervision process.

My main challenge was becoming familiar with the book and the OTIPM as it was not a model I had used myself in practice. I had to work through the steps with the students in the occupational therapy process, learning as I went along, but also making sure I assigned the reading in time to help students prepare for the next step. I wanted them to always be ready for the weekly discussion and I liked that it gave me an understanding of what we were going to talk about so that I felt prepared. This may also relate to my own developing confidence in the long-arm supervisor role. The book was a comfort to me as it provided a process I could clearly follow with the students. In retrospect, perhaps I could have been less directive at times and let students work to their own pace but I think this may have made our discussions less rich.

Supporting students on role-emerging placements often presents us as educators with complex and challenging situations. The book went some way to helping meet those challenges through providing guidance for the supervision process. Another crucial point was the support I received from other long-arm supervisors. If I had a question I could contact Dr. Kennedy-Behr or the university's placement coordinator. This helped me validate my own supervisory process.

The book in addition to providing me with a structure, also supported the discussions I had with the students about their reasoning. It is a challenge for a long-arm supervisor to assess students' abilities when we cannot be always on-site to observe them. Hence, we must rely on what the students share with us and listen to their perspectives. Our discussions on the activities in the book enabled me to gather some information for their evaluations.

Both students felt that the book was a useful tool for structuring supervision. They also commented on how using the structured guidance of the OTIPM could have enhanced their understanding of the occupational therapy process in earlier placements. From my perspective, I think that the book would make supervision more uniform by providing a clear tool to elicit reasoning among students in practice learning throughout their education.

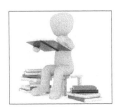

PRACTICAL TIPS
....

1   As a long-arm supervisor, be prepared to spend time becoming familiar with the contents of the book so that you can assign the correct chapters for the students to focus on at the right time during the placement.
2   When students have specific questions about the occupational therapy process, they can be redirected to the book.
3   Set up your own supportive networks so that you can discuss and share your successes and challenges with other educators.
4   Think about using the book as part of a pre-placement education programme for educators (often run as part of a university program).

CHAPTER SUMMARY

This book in draft form has been used in settings without traditional occupational therapy roles in the United Kingdom, Australia, Vanuatu and Canada. The book supported educators in their role by providing an extra resource, making sure everyone was 'on the same page' and providing a standardised way of conveying information about the occupational therapy process. The book was also useful in supporting students in their ability to apply theory to practice, however some contextualisation was needed for different settings. Student feedback about the book was positive in all settings, indicating a potential for the book to be used internationally.

REFERENCES

Dancza KM (2015) *Structure and uncertainty: The 'just right' balance for occupational therapy student learning on role-emerging placements in schools*. Doctor of Philosophy, The University of Queensland, Queensland, Australia.

Dancza KM, Copley J, Rodger S, Moran M (2016) 'The development of a theory-informed workbook as an additional support for students on role-emerging placements'. *British Journal of Occupational Therapy*, 79(4), 235–243.

De Bono E (1985) *Six Thinking Hats: An essential approach to business management*. London, UK: Little, Brown and Company.

Fisher AG (2009) *Occupational therapy intervention process model: A model for planning and implementing top-down, client centred, and occupation-based interventions.* Fort Collins, CO: Three Star Press.

Pidgeon F (2015) 'Occupational therapy: What does this look like practised in very remote indigenous areas?'. *Rural and Remote Health, 15*(2), 3002.

Townsend EA, Polatajko HJ, eds (2013) *Enabling occupation II: Advancing an occupational therapy vision for health, well-being, and justice through occupation.* 2nd edn. Ottawa, ON: Canadian Association of Occupational Therapists Publications ACE.

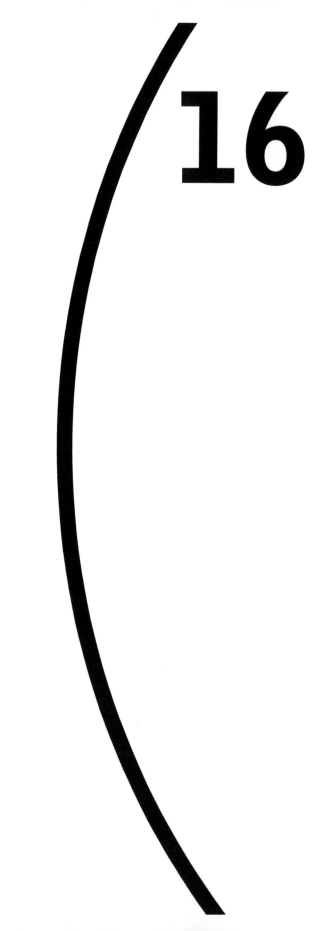

16

CHAPTER 16
CASE STUDIES IN ROLE-ESTABLISHED PLACEMENT SETTINGS
Sarah Harvey, Sarah E. Cullen and Anita Volkert

INTENDED CHAPTER OUTCOMES

By the end of this chapter, readers will have an overview of:

- The implementation of this book in role-established placement settings, namely in a child and adolescent mental health service, in an inpatient hospital setting, and a comparison of a role-established dementia care placement with a role-emerging placement in a school setting
- Issues and themes that emerged from having students on placement using the occupation-centred concepts presented in this book
- Practical tips and advice for implementing the occupation-centred structure presented in this book in similar settings

INTRODUCTION

This chapter reflects how this book (in draft form) and the Occupational Therapy Intervention Process Model (OTIPM; Fisher, 2009) have been applied in settings with an established occupational therapy role and service. Three case studies are presented to illustrate the experiences of educators and students.

The first case study (case study 4) outlines how this occupation-centred structure was used to guide student placements in a dementia care service in the United Kingdom. Interestingly, the author of this case study describes how she simultaneously used the book on role-established and role-emerging placements and contrasts the learning from both experiences. The second case study (case study 5) presents how this book was used to develop an occupational therapy service and student placements in an inpatient child and adolescent mental health service in the United Kingdom. The final case study (case study 6) shares the experiences of occupational therapists in two inpatient hospital settings in Australia.

CASE STUDY 4: UNITED KINGDOM ROLE-ESTABLISHED PLACEMENT IN A DEMENTIA CARE SERVICE COMPARED WITH A ROLE-EMERGING SCHOOL-BASED PLACEMENT (SARAH HARVEY)

CONTEXT

At the time of using a draft version of this book, I (Sarah Harvey) was working part-time as an occupational therapist in a specialist dementia care service within the National Health Service and part-time as a senior lecturer in occupational therapy. The specialist dementia care service was based in the community with a multidisciplinary team that consisted of two community psychiatric nurses, two support workers, one psychology assistant and two occupational therapists. Most of the work took place in the individual's homes or care (residential) homes. The service operated a shared caseload model; the client caseload was discussed at weekly team meetings, plans were agreed and tasks delegated.

At the same time, I was a part-time occupational therapy lecturer and part of my role was to provide long-arm supervision. I supervised several students on role-emerging placements within specialist and non-specialist school settings. It was during this process of supervising students in parallel, in both settings, that I started to appreciate the value of the book structure for both placement contexts. All the students were having to work without direct supervision for some part of the week. What I found most interesting were the comparisons I made between the learning generated by the students in each setting at the same point of their placement.

I found the book particularly helpful to guide the students through the occupational therapy process. It prompted students to think, try things out for themselves and to begin to make their own decisions about their practice. It allowed them to be more independent outside the supervision boundaries. Within the long-arm supervisory role, it also offered me a structure to follow which kept me on task and ultimately occupation-centred. The following sections are my own reflections about the placements and the insights I gained. There are many who helped me shape my learning and in particular I would like to thank Vicki Wells for her contribution.

AUTONOMY VERSES CONFORMITY AND DEPENDENCE

Within the long-arm supervision role, the students were being challenged from the start to consider the occupational therapy process in its raw form: formulating rapport with the team, thinking about the value of occupational therapy in the service and marketing their worth. These tasks almost forced students to think for themselves as the answers were not there in the form of an established occupational therapy role and service.

In comparison, the students on the role-established placement had all this laid out for them: the team was established, the structure was in place, the multidisciplinary relationships

Table 16.1 Differences between placement structures which influenced students' questions

Role-emerging	Role-established
The students had to consider the occupational therapy role within the service. They needed to ask themselves "what do I have to offer that is unique?"	The students were told about the service and observed and replicated what the occupational therapist did.
The students had to identify referral criteria and how to prioritise their caseloads.	The students attended a referral meeting and the occupational therapist was allocated a referral, which was passed on to the students.
The students had to consider the client context and liaise with relevant professionals, staff and families to establish suitable assessment processes.	The students observed the occupational therapist arranging the assessment within an established procedure and shadowed the therapist undertaking the assessment.
The students had to consider appropriate documentation/confidentiality and appropriate storage of notes.	The students accessed the notes on the electronic database and followed established protocols.

formed and the generic assessment process formulated. When comparing the students' experiences between role-established and role-emerging placements, I felt the role-established placement structure encouraged students to conform unquestioningly to the role and become dependent on the occupational therapists to model what they were expected to do. In the role-emerging placement, students asked "what shall we do and why?" while in the role-established placement students asked, "when shall we do it and how?"

I did not believe the difference in the students' approach was a reflection on the students' abilities; instead I felt they were encouraged by the nature of the placement culture and expectations. Table 16.1 illustrates how I thought the placements differed for the students.

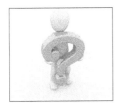

PRACTICAL TIPS

When thinking about your role as an educator in role-established or role-emerging placements, consider:

1   Are students asking "what shall we do and why?" or "when shall we do it and how?"

2 What do you think is influencing this? (Consider your own supervision style, the team's interactions with the students, the organisational structures and procedures etc.)

3 Can you identify the enablers and barriers to the students' learning in your team?

FOLLOWING IN AN OCCUPATIONAL THERAPISTS' FOOTSTEPS: DO OCCUPATIONAL THERAPY STUDENTS NEED TO STEP IN LINE?

I remember when I first trained as a practice educator and how I attempted to provide an up-to-date student file which outlined every part of the service provision and what the student had to do. Whist this had many benefits and is something which is encouraged in Chapter 5, I also reflected on how the students on placement may interpret this information.

In my experience, students' immediate default behaviour is to try and fit in on placement. I observed students doing this through mirroring the activity that was prevalent within the team: they would observe and then administer the generic assessments used, they would co-facilitate a pre-written group session and generally replicate what I and other staff members were doing.

Whilst I encouraged the students' willingness to fit in and engage in the normal process of the team, I questioned whether this process was the best learning experience for them. By encouraging this we were suggesting that students should adhere to procedures without thought, which seemed to be dismissing the students' developing occupational therapy skills and learning they brought from university.

When I saw students in a role-emerging placement setting alongside a role-established placement setting I discovered how valuable the students' fresh look at the situation could be (in the role-emerging placement). I saw the benefits of the students' 'clean sheet' perspective and how these ideas opened channels of creative solutions.

I have learnt from my experience in the lecture room that students want you to give them the answers, but as soon as they have the answer they no longer think (if indeed there is an ultimate answer). The most frustrating and anxiety-provoking position for a student is not knowing. As occupational therapists, we do not always have the answer and on qualifying we don't have someone providing solutions, so I feel that the sooner students can think through uncertainty and flex their autonomous muscles the better.

When working as an occupational therapist with clients, I would encourage people to come up with their own solutions. In contrast, as an educator, I often felt that I should provide all the answers without allowing students to find out for themselves.

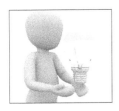

PRACTICAL TIPS
....

1   Reflect on the questions in Table 16.1. Which questions more closely reflect what your students are asking?
2   In a role-established setting, to prompt students to think about the occupational therapy role for themselves, adopt a position of curiosity and perhaps even offer your service some fresh perspectives, try using the questions in Table 16.2.

Table 16.2 Aligning the level of thinking required between role-established and role-emerging placements

Role-established scenario	Prompt questions
The students were told about the service and observed and replicated what the occupational therapist did.	Ask the student to consider the occupational therapy role within the service: – What is the need in the local area? – What do policy and guidelines recommend for this group of people? – What can occupational therapy offer? – What else could the service offer if there were no barriers?
The students attended a referral meeting and the occupational therapist was allocated a referral, which was passed on to the students.	– Why do you think we have these referral criteria? Consider the service's policy and service expectations. – Why do you think we've received that referral? – Does it meet our service criteria? – How quickly do I need to see them? – Who is the most appropriate person to allocate that to? Why? – What form of assessment should I use?
The students observed the occupational therapist arranging the assessment within an established procedure and shadowed the therapist undertaking the assessment.	– Consider why this assessment has been chosen, what information am I trying to gather and why? – What other assessment have you seen that could be appropriate to use? – Is this assessment process occupationally focused? If not how would you improve it?
The students accessed the notes on the electronic database and followed established protocols.	– What policies do you have to adhere to when documenting information and why? – What do you think are the best ways of documenting what we have seen? – What recommendations would you make? – Could we improve our documentation process? If so, how?

WHEN OCCUPATION IS OUT OF FOCUS

I have been in the humbling position of transferring from occupational therapy practitioner to occupational therapy lecturer. Whilst the students enjoyed my up-to-date clinical practice examples, on reflection I felt that the organisational pressures experienced in the workplace had smudged my occupational focus. Whilst using this book with students on placement I could challenge and consolidate a lot of my practice and make sure I was implementing and encouraging a truly top-down, occupation-centred approach.

In some teams I have worked in, occupational therapists and other disciplines within the team were expected to work as generic team members. The impact this had on my practice was that the occupation or 'doing' was not always at the centre of my practice. It factored in observations, it was reflected in my treatment plans and it was very much in the framework in my mind, but somehow some of the everyday tasks of crises management detracted from my occupation-centred work.

In my discussion with other occupational therapists, it appeared that I was not alone in these challenges. Some of my colleagues reflected that they were not always productively working with their caseload in an occupation-centred way; instead they felt they were firefighting. They gave examples of constant risk management and crisis intervention. When students were introduced to this fast-paced environment with crisis after crisis, it was difficult for them to work out what was the occupational therapy role. They often observed, for example, the occupational therapists assist in hospital admissions and being allocated to crisis work to minimise risk.

Thus, within a 'skill share' session (peer support and education) we looked at the OTIPM and reflected on our work. We discovered some interesting findings which we summarised as follows:

- We felt there was an over-reliance on client self-reporting with limited client observation.
- Time restrictions reduced the ability to re-evaluate outcomes in an occupation-centred way (so we had little idea about the ongoing effectiveness of our interventions).
- Interventions were not occupation-centred, and were instead service-driven, e.g. the goal was discharge rather than client priority to re-engage in occupations of meaning to them.
- There was a prominent focus on physical health and risk management, not occupational well-being.

The group felt somewhat disillusioned with the service and their ability to use their occupation-centred perspective. Through our discussions and by using the OTIPM within team supervision sessions, the occupational therapists could reflect on their work and consider good examples of practice and ways of re-focusing on occupation. My peers were genuinely excited about this return to occupation, believing this approach a useful way to get back to the roots of occupational therapy, enhance the service for clients and affirm their role within the team.

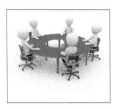

PRACTICAL TIPS

1   Students can provide a valuable opportunity to open a dialogue within a team about current practices and potential for service improvements. Learning from and with students can begin this process. Questions which I found useful as a way of reflecting on my practice included:
    –   How can I create opportunities to listen to students and remain open to challenges from students?
    –   Do I ask the students to provide feedback on what they have observed about the team?
    –   Do I ask the students for feedback on my own performance?
    –   How comfortable do I feel about asking students for this feedback? Why?
    –   What could I do differently?
2   To find out more from the students' perspectives, I found the following conversation starters useful:
    –   What are you learning from university and how is it similar or different from what you are seeing in practice?
    –   What are your expectations about the service?
    –   What might you offer if there were not any barriers? What might the service look like? What would be an 'ideal' scenario?
    –   Are there any creative solutions that you could suggest?

OCCUPATIONAL PERFORMANCE ANALYSIS VERSES GENERIC ASSESSMENT

If my colleagues felt that the occupational focus of their work had shifted to a generic focus, I wondered how this was impacting on how occupational therapy students understood their role on placement. It was not surprising that students reported a lack of clarity of the occupational therapy role when they were in a team of professionals completing the same job roles (generic team working). The following example helped me to see how easy it was for students to lose their occupational therapy focus.

The dementia services team members were trained in the use of dementia care mapping (Brooker and Surr, 2005). Dementia care mapping is a tool that maps a person's behaviour, what a person is doing, and his/her mood and engagement every five minutes. It gives a value against how engaged a person is and whether his/her mood is positive or negative. It also records the quality of interactions when a member of staff interacts with an individual (Brooker and Surr, 2005). Whilst this tool maps what the person is doing and his/her mood at the time, it doesn't detail how he/she are completing their occupations.

On one occasion, the team had been referred a lady (we will call her 'Pat', which is not her real name) who was reported to be very disruptive within the care home environment. She was behaving in an agitated way throughout the day, she would constantly be in and out of everyone's rooms, she would often try and leave the home, and she would complain that someone had stolen her money. Pat used to enjoy playing Bingo but had recently been too agitated to engage in this activity.

The team agreed that it would be useful to conduct a dementia care mapping assessment with Pat while she was involved in a Bingo game. My occupational therapy student asked to go along and observe with the team member (not an occupational therapist). My student was keen to learn about the dementia care mapping tool and had read the manual and wanted to observe using this framework. As an occupational therapist, I too had been enchanted by this standardised tool and had trained to administer it. However, I wanted to see if the student would remain more closely focused on occupation if she used an occupational performance analysis (see Chapter 8) to guide her observations instead of the dementia mapping tool. I think initially the student was disappointed as she wanted to try out the standardised generic assessment utilised by the team.

During the observation using the dementia care mapping tool, the team identified that Bingo had a positive impact on Pat's mood and that she remained more settled when playing it. However, by using the occupational performance analysis tool the occupational therapy student had been able to identify the problems Pat faced as she engaged with the task and changes that needed to take place to make her engagement in the activity more successful. These are summarised in Table 16.3

Table 16.3 Analysis of 'Pat' playing Bingo using an occupational performance analysis

Summary of the student's observations:

- Pat looked for a long time at another resident pacing the room and then asked the facilitator which numbers he had called out.
- Pat made comments about a resident pacing the room interrupting her playing Bingo.
- Pat required prompts to tick off her missed numbers.
- Pat looked out the window several times.
- Pat did not call 'Bingo' when all her numbers were covered.
- The environment was noisy, there was lots of movement in the room, people walked in and out, and the noise of the cutlery and crockery being set for dinner was loud from the adjoining room.

Summary of the recommendations made:

- Education: a workshop for residential care home staff members (including the Bingo facilitator) on how to enhance the occupations of residents, including changing the way the Bingo numbers are called and reinforcement which could be offered to keep people on task.
- Compensation: environmental change, suggesting Pat sit nearer to the facilitator and away from the window and view of lounge, to reduce distractions and promote hearing.
- Change time of the activity to limit noise of dinner preparations.

This experience highlighted for the student and the wider team the unique occupational focus which occupational therapy provides. The team found this particularly useful as an illustration of the occupational therapy role. Moreover, the occupational therapists appreciated the clear example of how their unique perspective can enhance the work of the generic team.

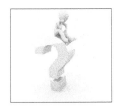

PRACTICAL TIPS

Some questions that I have found useful to help me reflect on my practice and service:

1   Does the assessment I use assess the occupational performance of the person?
2   Is my intervention focused on enhancing the person's occupations?
3   Is there anything I could change within my team assessment to help me gather occupationally focused information?
4   Is there anything I could change in the way I deliver my interventions that would promote occupations being performed in context?

CASE STUDY 5: UNITED KINGDOM ROLE-ESTABLISHED PLACEMENT IN AN INPATIENT CHILD AND ADOLESCENT MENTAL HEALTH UNIT (SARAH CULLEN)

CONTEXT

Since I graduated with my Master's degree in Occupational Therapy in Ireland, I (Sarah Cullen) have always been interested in working as an occupational therapist with children and adolescents accessing mental health services. Prior to training as an occupational therapist, I worked with adolescents in care settings in the United States. I was therefore keen to undertake a role in England in an inpatient secure mental health setting for young people.

The service was managed by a private health care provider commissioned to admit clients who could not be successfully placed elsewhere due to their presenting needs. The clients had symptoms relating to trauma, anxiety, depression, psychosis, disorders of conduct and emotion, autistic spectrum disorder and attention deficit hyperactivity disorder. The young people were considered to be a risk to themselves and others and were in detention under the Mental Health Act (Department of Health, 1983) in the secure hospital environment. The service provided medical, therapeutic and educational input via a team comprising of psychiatrists, nurses and support workers, psychologists, family therapists, speech and language therapists, an occupational therapist, and teachers. The service had three wards: an acute admissions ward, a recovery and rehabilitation ward, and a step-down ward outside of the secure perimeter.

I was employed as the principal occupational therapist and I was also managing three occupational therapy assistants. Due to the complexities involved in establishing a new occupational therapy service (my post had been vacant for over a year), I quickly became aware that I needed my own support to develop my role. I secured external supervision from an experienced university-based occupational therapist, who introduced me to the OTIPM and a draft version of this book to help guide my practice. From my experiences of using the OTIPM for my own practice, as well as to guide occupational therapy student placements, some key learning emerged.

FEELING ISOLATED AS THE SOLE QUALIFIED OCCUPATIONAL THERAPIST

My priority when I started my job was to establish the occupational therapy role within the multidisciplinary treatment pathway. I wanted to feel confident in my reasoning first, before I attempted to assert and clarify the role of occupational therapy to the team. This was particularly important as the team had not had an occupational therapist in post for over a year and they had a wide range of expectations for what I would do.

I was experienced at using theoretical models of practice such as the Canadian Model of Occupational Performance and Engagement (CMOP-E; Townsend and Polatajko, 2007) and the Model of Human Occupation (MOHO; Kielhofner, 2008), however I did not find that these models were sufficient on their own when establishing the occupational therapy process.

I developed my knowledge of the OTIPM through trying out the steps in my practice and reflecting on these experiences. I would have liked to learn about the model through working alongside another occupational therapist who was using it; however, I did not find another occupational therapist using the model and my impression at the time was that there was little openness to consider another model in mental health practice other than the MOHO (Kielhofner, 2008). While I had found the MOHO useful for some assessments and interventions, I became frustrated as I did not find that the occupational therapy process in the MOHO provided me with enough guidance to enact my practice and to remain occupation-centred.

Having the support of an external occupational therapy supervisor was critical to guide me and clarify my reasoning. In my initial supervision sessions, I was bringing along 'therapy programmes' which I had read about in the literature or seen other occupational therapists use in mental health settings. I was focused on the tasks I had to complete (such as developing the service's activity schedule and monitoring the work of the occupational therapy assistants), but without thinking about the ultimate purpose of occupational therapy in the setting. Time in supervision allowed me to explore *what* I was doing and more importantly *why* I was doing it.

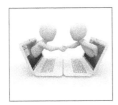

PRACTICAL TIPS

1   Working in a setting as the only occupational therapist can be a daunting experience. It does, however, offer many opportunities to try things out and work in a way which is not constrained by existing service structures. If you have no occupational therapy supervision in your setting, seek it out elsewhere through a different service or university. Time spent in supervision is well worth it as it will keep you on task, foster a sense of job satisfaction and ultimately enable you to provide a better occupational therapy service for your clients.
2   The occupation-centred principles presented in this book are useful not only for student practice learning, but also for occupational therapists who are developing a service or working as a sole clinician. They can also be used to structure supervision or mentoring of occupational therapists.

TAKING OCCUPATIONAL THERAPY STUDENTS WHEN THE SERVICE WAS STILL DEVELOPING

The service wanted me to take occupational therapy students on placement as it was a marker of quality provision. Initially, the thought of establishing student placements seemed like it was a longer-term plan. I did not think I would have capacity for students due to my caseload and clinical governance responsibilities. I was concerned that the service would not be developed enough to role model a well-functioning service for students. I also felt that I needed to have more knowledge and competence with regards to using the OTIPM before I could explain it to someone else. However, I later came to realise that the setting offered learning opportunities like a role-emerging placement and that I could learn alongside the students. I even found explaining my developing understanding of the OTIPM actually helped my own learning.

In conjunction with the university, the placement was established as a 2:1 model (two students to one educator), with third (final) year occupational therapy students. I thought that by having two students together they would be able to work jointly on projects and offer additional peer support and learning. It also meant that I did not feel so pressured to be with the students all the time.

The draft version of this book (Dancza, 2015) was utilised during the students' placement and was of benefit to both the students and myself as educator, in terms of embedding occupation and seeing it applied in practice. I was familiar with the OTIPM as I had used it during my own supervision (with the university mentor) for about six months prior to the students' placement. I felt, however, that I was still learning and therefore the students and I both developed our knowledge together through applying techniques from the book.

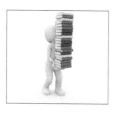

PRACTICAL TIPS

1   Try to be realistic; you do not need to showcase an 'ideal service'. There are many learning opportunities when there are challenges to be resolved. Joint problem solving with students allows them to develop their own reasoning skills. They can also offer useful new perspectives for the service.

2   Remember that as a role model to students, it is important to demonstrate your willingness to identify gaps in your own knowledge and to continuously learn. Consider allocating one learning objective to a project which involves the students and educator learning together, perhaps focusing on an area you have identified for your own continuous professional development (CPD).

3   Consider what currently works well and what you would like to change in your service. Having students on placement may be one way of progressing a project. Students can make excellent team members, contributing their up-to-date knowledge and fresh approaches.

PERCEPTIONS AND EXPECTATIONS OF THE MULTIDISCIPLINARY TEAM

Prior to starting as the principal occupational therapist, the occupational therapy assistants worked as activity coordinators who were managed by the nursing team. I found one of the main challenges to re-establishing occupational therapy in the service was the disparate understanding and expectations of my role (and the new occupational therapy assistants) from the multidisciplinary team.

I initially attempted to address this by providing education (telling people what I did) to the team members. Unfortunately, this did not have the desired impact. So, I began to question:

–   Why did I think the team's perceptions and expectations needed to be addressed?
–   What were my feelings about the team's understanding of the occupational therapy role?
–   Was a teaching method the best approach to use?

Early on in their placement the students also identified the multidisciplinary team's perceptions and expectations of occupational therapy as a challenge. They were keen to create a leaflet about the role of occupational therapy to disseminate throughout the team. I recognised from my own experience as a student that this is the 'go-to' method to increase awareness of something (like my thinking that telling people about my role would improve understanding).

I encouraged the students to consider the same questions I had asked myself. We were then able to discuss these ideas, as well as my own experiences with similar struggles. I shared with the students how I thought I may be more successful in educating the team by spending that time delivering occupational therapy with the occupational therapy assistants. The team learned about occupational therapy from what I showed them occupational therapists do. This, along with explaining my reasoning for what I was doing, was successful and the team did eventually shift in their expectations about my role and valued my contributions.

Enabling others to observe our practice to see and learn about the occupational therapy role worked well to educate the nursing team, support workers and therapy team. However, it did not address the prescriptive requests from hospital managers and doctors who did not have the opportunity to observe occupational therapy practice on a regular basis. I needed a different approach. For these interactions, which tended to be via email or in meetings, I found it was beneficial to thank the professionals for their input and then ask why they were seeking that input. I asked questions such as:

– When is this most challenging for the young person?
– What occupations is this impacting on?
– What would a good outcome be? What would you notice is different?

This line of questioning enabled me to better understand what they were hoping to achieve and it helped me to focus on the occupations which were of most concern. This reinforced that my focus was on occupation and provided me with a logical starting point to begin my occupation-centred occupational therapy process.

I found that how we 'market' our occupational therapy role makes a significant difference to how we are perceived in the multidisciplinary team. When we reinforced our role only through labelling our interventions on a timetable (e.g. newspaper group, social interaction group, games group), we communicate that we facilitate activities and not occupations which are meaningful to the client (Cullen and Warren, 2013). This provides a limited view as to the value of occupational therapy. Using the activities within this book and the guidance of the OTIPM developed my own confidence in my professional identity and enabled me to support students develop an occupation-centred approach.

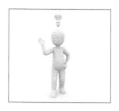

PRACTICAL TIPS

1   Try using coaching strategies (such as those suggested in the Professional Learning through Useful Support Framework in Chapter 14) to help students identify the knowledge they possess and the role they have in championing the direction of occupational therapy in the future. Supporting students' development of reasoning skills (as opposed to learning 'patterns' of what occupational therapists do) is key.
2   When working to improve the multidisciplinary team's understanding of occupational therapy, I found the following questions helpful:
    –   Why do I want to improve the team's understanding? Will the time spent increasing awareness have a direct impact on client care? Am I concerned about this because I feel frustrated and under-valued within a team? Would improving the team's understanding be an effective method to address this?
    –   Why might colleagues be prescriptive about what they want from occupational therapy? Is occupational therapy susceptible to this because we often work within a medical model of health care delivery? Is there anything I could be doing differently?

A TIMELINE TO PACE THE PLACEMENT

The students and I often referred to the placement timeline in the book (see Figure 5.1 in Chapter 5) to help identify priorities for each week. The placement timeline was also useful to clearly outline the differing pace of the occupational therapy process in this setting. Most notable was the longer time required for students to understand the setting, build rapport with clients and prioritise occupational needs than they had previously experienced.

An early focus for students was on the self-reflection checklist (see Chapter 5). Identifying their learning preferences from the beginning addressed potential rivalry amongst the students, as the differences were acknowledged and the benefits and challenges of both characteristics were highlighted. For example, with my students, one student's strength was being self-directed and enthusiastic whilst the other's strength was knowing his/her limitations and recognising his/her learning needs. The contrasting styles benefited both learners once they identified them and discussed them openly.

Students had the opportunity to assess clients during their placement using the occupational performance analysis examples as a guide (see Chapter 8). During the observations, students made their own notes and later translated these onto the occupational performance analysis form. The students assisted each other by verbally presenting a draft version of the occupational performance analysis which enabled them to learn from each other and identify gaps in their information. While this format took students time to learn, by following this guidance they developed their observational skills and highlighted useful information for intervention planning.

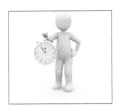

PRACTICAL TIPS

1   Prepare with the students a realistic timeline of what is achievable during placement. The placement timeline contained in the book is a useful tool which can be adapted. Remember that students will be nervous and enthusiastic, as we would be with a new job, and structure for the first week is invaluable as a foundation for the remainder of the placement.
2   It is sometimes helpful to discuss with students that learning new concepts and using theory to inform their practice is a complex and demanding challenge. It takes time and effort and while progress can seem slow, it is important that they read, discuss, experiment and reflect to enhance their understanding of what it means to be an occupational therapist.

CASE STUDY 6: AUSTRALIAN ROLE-ESTABLISHED PLACEMENTS IN INPATIENT HOSPITAL SERVICES (ANITA VOLKERT)

CONTEXT

At the time of using this book in draft form, I (Anita Volkert) was working as a lecturer and placements coordinator within occupational therapy education in Australia. My colleagues, Michelle Wykes and Monica Vasquez, used this resource to direct placements in their respective hospital sites. Both sites were large general hospitals situated in urban settings, providing general admissions and specialist services (e.g. neurological rehabilitation, oncology). Occupational therapy services were ward- and/or outpatient-based and situated within multidisciplinary contexts. Teams included medicine, nursing, physiotherapy, some access to speech pathology, radiography, social work, and both general and allied health assistant workers. The occupational therapy role, whilst well-defined, was restricted by the setting's priorities (as will be described later in this case study).

Both sites were experimenting with alternative models of placement, such as peer mentoring (Penman and Ratz, 2015), to increase placement capacity and decrease supervisory burden. This meant that students were starting to work with less direct supervision (Health Education Training Institute, 2015), which was an unfamiliar experience for the educators in these settings.

Both educators felt that the use of the book assisted students to move from a purely procedural approach to practice learning – where they asked for constant direction in what to do, what was required to pass, or wanting to copy from their supervisor – to an approach where they paused, tried to think for themselves and reflected on their actions. The OTIPM was considered useful and highly relevant to the settings, particularly due to its highly procedural and process-driven nature. Moreover, both educators had some familiarity with it prior to using it during this placement.

While the hospital setting is usually regarded as a traditional placement setting with close supervision available to students, both educators pointed out that occupational therapists in these settings have a high caseload and are juggling multiple demands throughout the day. With the need to leave students to operate as independently as possible, the settings had more in common with less traditional, role-emerging settings than was first apparent.

THE INHERENT PRACTICE RESTRICTIONS WITHIN THE HOSPITAL SETTING

There are several inherent practice restrictions with the hospital setting which challenged the students' use of this book in this context. For example, an acute hospital places emphasis on a client's body functions and structures, diagnosis or health condition as causative of the challenges experienced in occupational performance. Students found it difficult to reconcile their learning about the impact of multiple factors on occupational performance (as described in many models of occupational therapy practice, including the OTIPM), when many of the assessment tools they are exposed to focused only on a person's impairment.

Another example of an inherent restriction of the setting was in the choice of occupations that students could focus on. In these settings, there is an emphasis on one domain of occupation, that of self-care. Therefore, while students understood the importance of client choice in occupations, the emphasis was necessarily placed on self-care.

One perhaps more subtle restriction students discovered in the hospital setting was not being able to take notes while observing. The guidance in the book recommends notes should be taken to aid memory. In some cases taking notes was prohibited due to infection control restrictions, where no materials can be taken into the client space. One educator commented that these restrictions and the speed of work required in the acute environment, might mean that there is no ability to take notes during a session, or even write them up immediately afterward. Whilst not ideal, this represents a reality of practice and therefore the skill of retaining information was critical for students to develop. These differences from the guidance provided in the book meant students required the contextualization of the information from educators to make best use of the resource. This requirement made sense when I considered it from a learning theory perspective (as introduced in Chapter 14).

Despite the challenges to implementing some of the concepts presented in this book, using the book also offered unexpected opportunities. One of the benefits of using this structure reported by the educators was that the students could explore different assessment tools which occupational therapists in the setting had little time to do. This enabled the educators to consider some of their own working practices and the potential for changes to improve service provision.

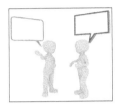

PRACTICAL TIPS

1 Reinforce for students that being in hospital is a person's context for a period. Enabling their occupations in this context will have an impact on the client's health and well-being and can assist in their recovery process.
2 Early in the placement, discuss with students the available opportunities for them in the setting.
3 Provide students with examples of completed assessment forms and other types of documentation so they are clear about the expectations for the setting.

THE IMPORTANCE OF INTRODUCTIONS AND BUILDING RAPPORT

Due to the potentially limited time available to move through the occupational therapy process in a hospital setting, it was vital that students could introduce themselves and their role clearly and succinctly. One educator felt that unless students could do this adequately, they could achieve very little else. As part of learning to describe the occupational therapy role both educators liked the example of the presentation about occupational therapy (see Chapter 5) and planned to use a similar idea in future placements.

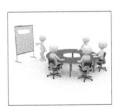

PRACTICAL TIPS

1 Encourage students to develop their own 'script' and presentation for introducing themselves, their role and the unique contribution of occupational therapy to clients, family and team members. This is to help them consolidate their own understanding and raise the profile of occupational therapy in the setting. Chapter 5 offers students some examples.
2 Create opportunities for students to present their role to others (such as in meetings, training events, information evenings etc.).

CREATING A SENSE OF OWNERSHIP

Educators felt that having contact details for team members – such as the physiotherapist, speech pathologist, social worker, or medical team – recorded in one place helped students navigate the often overwhelming and complex nature of the hospital environment. It was a way to give students a sense of ownership and control over the information they needed to gather to do their work and reduce their need to repeatedly ask their supervisor how to contact team members.

This brought up a key conversation about the difficulty educators who are on-site in a traditional placement may have in being able to judge when to step back and allow students some autonomy in their practice. On a role-emerging placement, that decision is taken out of their hands to some degree, as supervision is bounded and limited to specific times and days.

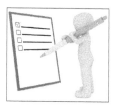

PRACTICAL TIPS

1   Reflect on the opportunities during the placement which encourage students' autonomy and decision making. Consider how minor changes, such as holding their own contact lists, could enhance students' independence.
2   Encourage students to follow the OTIPM and use their activity and occupational performance analysis tools during the placement, even when there are many competing pressures in the acute setting. As students are 'extras' in the setting, they can do some additional observations for their learning over and above what might be typical for the service and this can support them having a sense of ownership over their learning.

TENSION BETWEEN SERVICE DEMAND AND CLIENT-CENTREDNESS

Prioritisation was considered a critical skill for students to develop in the hospital setting. For example, students often experienced competing demands such as a family conference, a self-care assessment and two reviews to complete on any given morning. Students needed to know what to do first and how to manage their time so everything could be completed. The book offered lots of useful strategies to guide them to develop these complex skills (see Chapter 7).

In addition, the occupational therapy role was often externally set by the service, focusing on safe discharge and patient flow through. These priorities can at times be very different from the priorities an occupational therapist may choose in collaboration with a client if those service drivers were not present. Educators explained, however, that a discharge from hospital is a usually desired outcome for clients in this setting, along with a decrease in the occupational issues that either led to their admission or were interfering with their discharge (self-care, or getting around the home and community for example).

Different client and service priorities can present a confusing picture for students as they are developing their understanding of client-centred practice (also see a wider discussion of this in Chapter 11). This discrepancy was perhaps emphasised as students compared the occupational therapy process presented in the book with what they experienced in practice.

Balancing the need for discharge and patient flow with client-centredness is a complex area which creates tensions between the core philosophy of occupational therapy and the needs of the employing service for occupational therapists and students in the hospital setting. Students may need to refine their priority areas in accordance with the service, not just their preferences and the client's preferences. This was another unexpected opportunity for student learning as through using the book and comparing it with what was happening in practice (e.g. the dominance of the model, discharge is the measured outcome and client turnover is high), rich discussions were prompted.

As a profession, occupational therapy currently has a strong presence in the acute setting. However, our core philosophy, principles, knowledge and skills are already being used effectively in some areas in primary care and preventative approaches (for example, situated within GP surgeries/ambulance services to prevent admission, or working with populations to prevent ill-health through participation in occupation). Occupational therapists also work over periods of time with people with long-term disability and chronic conditions, to facilitate participation in occupations. Being open with students about these tensions and exploring when factors limit occupational therapy roles help students work within the realities of practice, whilst not limiting their understanding of their professional identity.

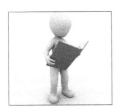

PRACTICAL TIPS

1   Encourage students to identify what occupations might be important for the client population. Help students focus on occupations, rather than tasks, and work through the possible tensions between the service demand of discharge and client choice.
2   The prioritisation exercises in the book (see Chapter 7) can help students consider their prioritisation process, explain their reasoning and justify their decisions (e.g. as preparation for ward meetings and case conferences).

CHAPTER SUMMARY

This chapter presented three case study illustrations of how this book (in draft form) and the OTIPM have been used in role-established placement settings. All three case studies highlighted some dissonance between occupation-centred practice and organisational expectations. The use of the OTIPM and this book supported staff members and students to see beyond the boundaries of the setting and conceptualise the broader practice possibilities of occupational therapy. The case studies explored examples of discussions that encouraged the students to provide a fresh look at service provision and gave practical tips on having creative conversations to consider future occupation-centred practice. This book could offer strategies to help occupational therapists resolve the tension that exists between service demands and client-centeredness for students and educators alike.

It is hoped that this chapter, and indeed the entire book, will give you an opportunity to reflect on your skills as an educator and become an expert facilitator. A key benefit of this book from an educator's perspective is using it as a tool to facilitate reasoning, to question what we do and why we do it and to mutually learn and develop our practice as occupation-centred occupational therapists. It is important that we re-evaluate how much information we deliver to students and when to hold back information to promote student discovery and learning. Overall, we hope that you will feel empowered to give students a voice in the profession and re-affirm your own occupation-centred philosophy.

REFERENCES

Brooker D, Surr C (2005) *Dementia care mapping: Principles and practice.* Bradford, UK: University of Bradford.

Cullen S, Warren A (2013) 'Reflecting on quality in an occupational therapy intellectual disability service'. *Irish Journal of Occupational Therapy,* 40(1), 3–10.

Dancza KM (2015) *Structure and uncertainty: The 'just right' balance for occupational therapy student learning on role-emerging placements in schools.* Doctor of Philosophy, The University of Queensland, Queensland, Australia.

Department of Health (1983) *Mental Health Act.* London, UK: Crown Copyright.

Fisher AG (2009) *Occupational therapy intervention process model: A model for planning and implementing top-down, client centred, and occupation-based interventions.* Fort Collins, CO: Three Star Press.

Health Education and Training Institute (2015–last update) *Report: Clinical placements in NSW.* Available: www.heti.nsw.gov.au/Global/ICTN/ICTN%20Forum%202014/

GOVERNMENT%20RELATIONS%20-%20Reporting%20-%20Clinical%20Placements%
20in%20NSW%202015%20-%20Full%20report.pdf [March 29, 2017].

Kielhofner G (2008) *A model of human occupation: Theory and application.* 4th edn. Baltimore, MD: Lippincott Williams & Wilkins.

Penman C, Ratz S (2015) 'A module-based approach to foster and document the intercultural process before and during the residence abroad'. *Intercultural Education, 26*(1), 49–61.

Townsend E, Polatajko HJ, eds (2007) *Enabling occupation II: Advancing an occupational therapy vision for health, well-being and justice through occupation.* Ottawa, ON: CAOT Publications ACE.

GLOSSARY

Activity: describes a general way in which something is done. Also described as 'task'.

Activity analysis: a process of breaking down an activity into the components that influence how it is chosen, organised and carried out within the environment to determine how it might be typically performed. Also described as 'task analysis'.

Client: a person or group who is accessing/receiving the services of occupational therapy (or other) personnel. Also described as 'patient', 'service user' or 'customer'. We also use the term 'person' interchangeably with 'client' when it is clear who is being discussed.

Educator: overarching term used to describe a person who provides guidance to students or less-experienced people within university or practice learning situations.

Long-arm supervisor: the occupational therapist who supervises and supports students, but who is not based at the placement site. Also described as 'fieldwork educator for independent community placements (FEICP)', 'off-site occupational therapist supervisor', 'occupational therapy practice placement educator, (OTPPE)', 'practice placement educator', 'off-site occupational therapist educator/supervisor' or 'off-site supervisor'.

Occupation: an (observable) activity which is done by a person such that it has individual meaning and purpose to that person.

Occupation-based: describes practice where the 'doing' of occupation is

the main ingredient in assessment, intervention and measure of outcomes.

Occupation-centred: the importance of occupation is central to assessment, intervention and evaluation. Enablement of occupation is the defining element. It is like 'task-orientated' or 'goal-orientated' approaches. Occupation-centred is made up of occupation-focused and occupation-based practice.

Occupation-focused: describes practice where information about the person, environment and occupation relates closely with occupational performance.

Occupational performance analysis: a structured and detailed way of observing a person performing an occupation in context to determine what is supporting or hindering him/her in being able to participate to his/her desired level.

Occupational profile: this is developed as we gather information about the occupational strengths, needs, wishes and circumstances of the person.

Occupational therapy: occupational therapists are concerned with how people 'occupy' their time. What people do to occupy their time (their occupations) is fundamental to their health and well-being. Daily life is made up of many occupations, such as getting ready to go out, cooking a meal or working. An occupational therapist will help people who may need support or advice if they are not able to do their occupations due to illness, disability, circumstances or because of changes in their lives as they get older.

Occupational Therapy Intervention Process Model (OTIPM): an occupational therapy professional reasoning model which is used in this book to guide occupation-centred practice.

On-site supervisor: non-occupational therapy personnel who supervises and supports students and who is based at the placement site. Also described as 'on-site associate supervisor', 'on-site practice placement educator (OSPPE)', 'primary supervisor' or 'agency staff member supervisor'.

Placement: the time students spend in authentic settings with people, where they have opportunities to consider person-occupation-environment relationships and the impact these have on people's health and well-being. Also described as 'fieldwork'.

Practice learning: the process of acquiring professional competence through experiences that are not bounded by time or place, with the guidance of more-experienced people.

Professional Learning through Useful Support (PLUS) Framework: an educational tool created to describe a set of guidance strategies used by skilled educators to support student practice learning, whilst acknowledging the critical influences of the practice and university contexts.

Project placement: where the student is in a setting with or without an established occupational therapy service with the primary intention of doing a piece of defined work.

Role-emerging placement: where the student is in a setting without an established occupational therapy service. Also described as 'alternative', 'non-traditional', 'a-typical', 'expanded', 'service-learning', or 'independent community' placement.

Role-established placement: where the student is in a setting with an on-site supervisor who holds an occupational therapy position. Also described as 'traditional' placement.

Supervisor: person who provides guidance to students or less-experienced people. Also described as 'clinical instructor', 'clinical educator', 'preceptor', 'practice educator', 'placement educator' or 'practice placement tutor'.

INDEX

Page numbers in *italic* indicate a figure and page numbers in **bold** indicate a table on the corresponding page.

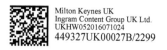

Milton Keynes UK
Ingram Content Group UK Ltd.
UKHW052016071024
449327UK00027B/2299